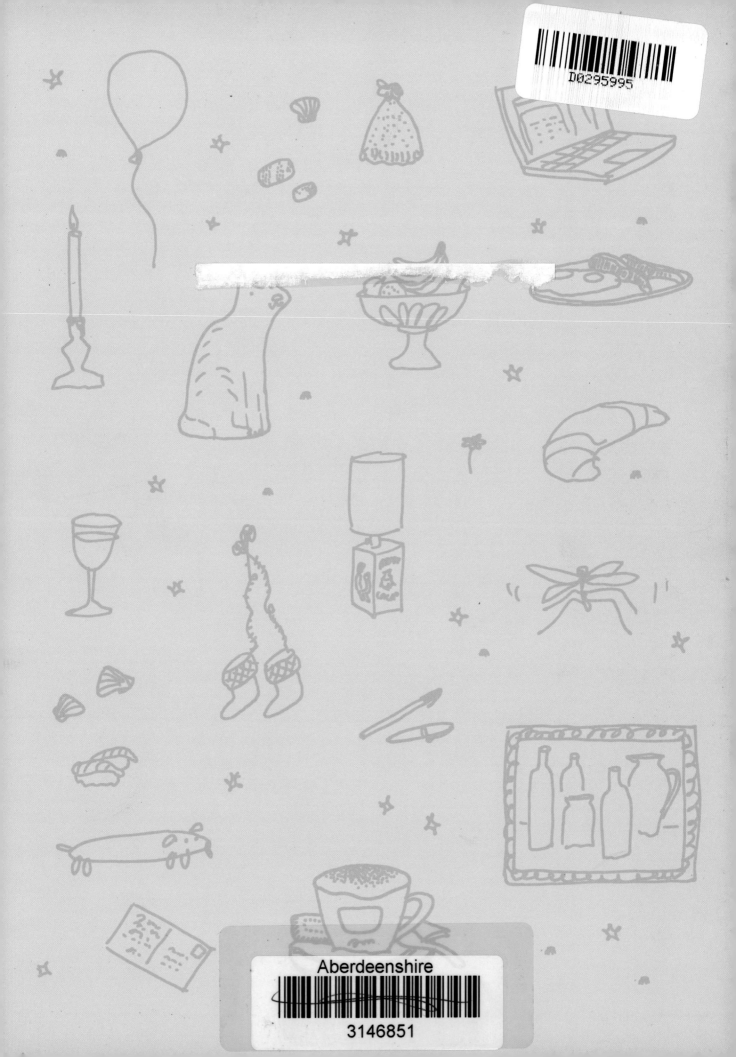

PROBABLY NOTHING

PROBABLY NOTHING

A diary of not-your-average nine months

Matilda Tristram

VIKING
an imprint of
PENGUIN BOOKS

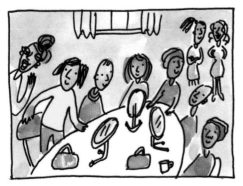

At the end of my treatment,
I go to a cancer patients'
make-over day.
'Can I get you a tea?'
'Oh yes please, milk,
no sugar.'

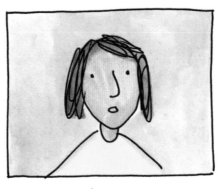

We introduce ourselves.
'I had surgery to remove
a tumour from my large
bowel back in February,
then 6 months of chemo.'

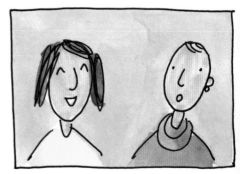

'And I was pregnant
at the same time.'
'Gosh, what a year!'

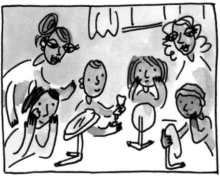

The make-up girls get us
to smear green stuff
all over our faces.
'A life-saver if you do
suffer from redness.'

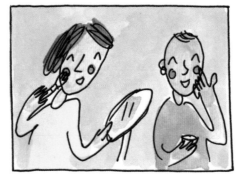

Then put blusher on.
'Should've just left holes
in the green stuff!'

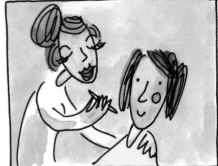

I enjoy pretending I don't
know how to do anything.
'Don't worry if you
don't feel confident
drawing eyebrows.'

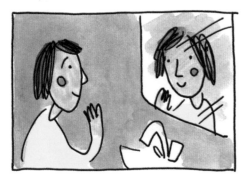

Go and inspect myself
in the loo, afterwards.
Surprisingly tasteful.
(Secretly I'd hoped they'd
make me look like Divine.)

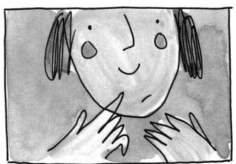

Want to celebrate the
proud return of my
one chin hair.

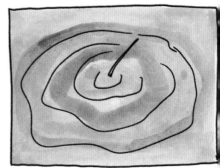

Resist drawing a
bull's eye round it with
everything in my
complimentary goodie bag.

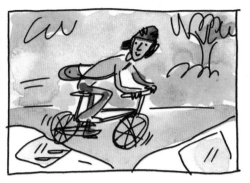

Cycle home, checking myself out in car windows every so often.

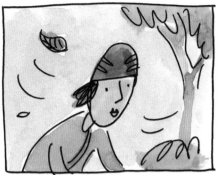

I try to go only on quiet roads. I'm more worried about being killed by stuff, these days.

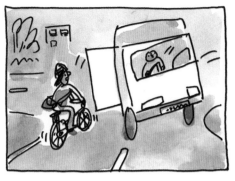

A van turns into the street I'm on. Its back door swings open and almost knocks me off my bike.

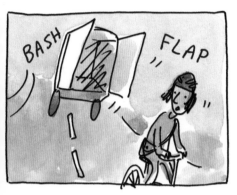

BASH

FLAP

Feel like the universe is still trying to get me.

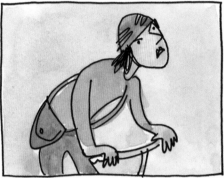

I want to shout: 'UNIVERSE, YOU WILL NOT GET ME!!'

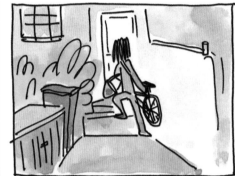

Make it home alive.

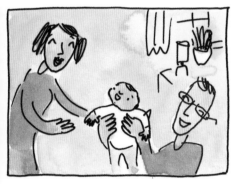

'Ooh! Look at Mummy!'

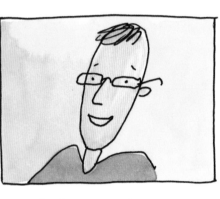

'Who is this glamorous woman?'

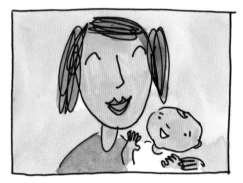

FEBRUARY

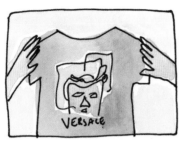

I was wearing my favourite T-shirt on the day of the diagnosis. I never want to wear it again.

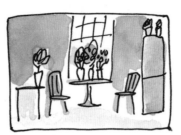

The flat is full of flowers.

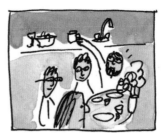

We all cram round our tiny kitchen table and start getting used to things. 'The great thing about your tiny kitchen is that I can reach anything without leaving my seat!'

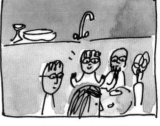

Mum tells us something about her PhD; 'It was the publisher who censored it, not the translator at all!'

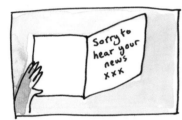

No one can bring themselves to write 'cancer' in a card.

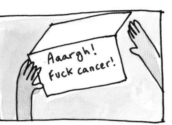

Apart from one friend who's had it before.

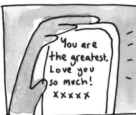

Lots of people send lovely messages.

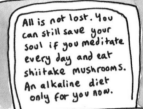

And not so lovely ones.

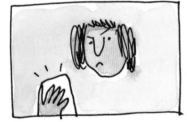

I get annoyed when people ask if they can pray for me. 'Do it if it makes you feel better!'

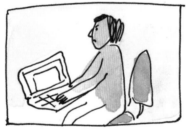

And when people I don't know very well ask me how I'm feeling. 'How do you fucking think I'm feeling!?'

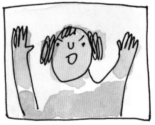

And when people send me emails about miracle cures. 'Lemon peel? Broccoli? I've been eating broccoli my entire life!'

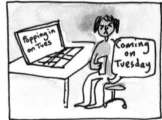

And when everyone wants to visit me all at once. 'I don't want to see ANYONE!'

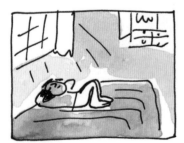

I lie on the bed in a patch of sun and remember lying on a rock by the sea at Point d'Endoume in Marseille.

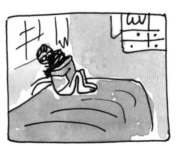

Me and Tom talk about the other holidays we'll go on and I cry.

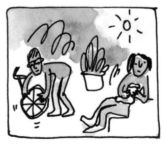

Tom fixes a tyre and I mend my slipper on the front step. It's good to be outside.

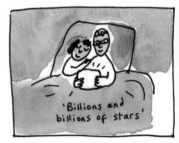

Brian Cox on the iPad helps me to fall asleep at night.

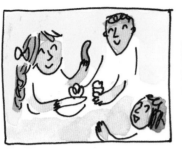

My friends, Mully and Cesca, come and visit. 'We brought you a plastic sausage!' 'And a plastic ice cream!' 'Oh! Thank you!'

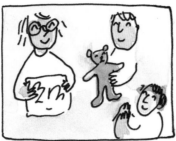

My aunts, Polly and Lucy, come and visit. 'We brought you a tapestry kit!' 'And a teddy!' 'Wonderful!'

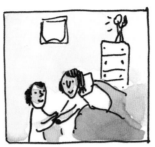

My sister, Hannah, comes and rubs arnica into my bruised hands (from the drip). 'If your hair falls out I'll get a number one in solidarity.'

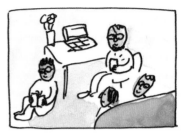

My step-dad, Mikey, wants to know about Twitter and everything starts to feel a bit more normal. 'So what is this, Tweety? Can I use it to message you?'

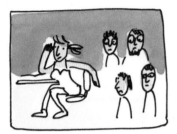

Then we go to see the oncologist and everything seems terrible again. 'We will give you chemotherapy but we can't be certain it will kill any remaining cancer cells.'

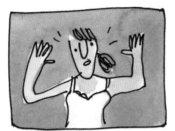

'We also don't know for certain if there are any cancer cells left! It's possible we got them all when we operated.'

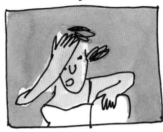

'As I see it, you've got three options; have chemo now and risk damaging the baby...'

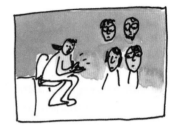

'...terminate the pregnancy and start chemo after that... and I must make you aware that chemo could make you infertile...'

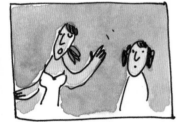

'Or delay treatment until after it's born.'

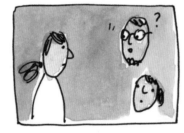

'The surgeon mentioned that as the cancer hasn't spread very far, there might be some sort of mild chemo available?'

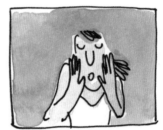

'Forgive me but the surgeon is not a cancer doctor.'

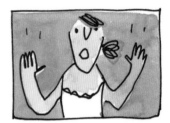

'Chemo is chemo. There is no such thing as mild chemotherapy. We need to attack you with it.' (I had asked her to 'Tell it to me straight'.)

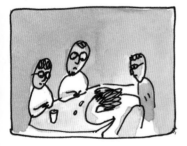

We sit in Costa for a bit and I bawl my eyes out. 'I don't want to do any of this!'

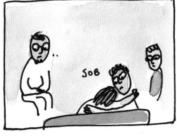

Then we go home and I bawl my eyes out some more. 'Well, whatever happens we'll make it work.'

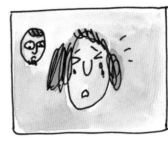

'We won't make it work if I'm dead!'

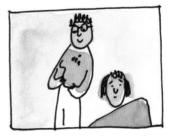

Mum says she's proud of my tears on her top and I feel slightly better.

Months ago I bought tickets for me and Tom to go up the Shard that evening.
We decide to go in spite of it all (it was his birthday).

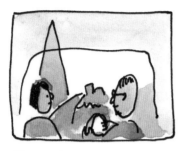

Mikey drives us as close as he can.
'I can see the appeal of living in London, so much fascinating stuff.'

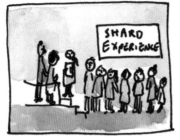

Long queue.
'I don't think I can stand up for that long.'
'Let's see if we can borrow a wheelchair.'

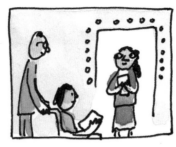

It was very revealing.
'Got this online reference.'
'Hello, Sir, do you have an online reference?'

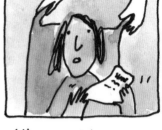

'Yes, me, I have an online reference!'
'Ah right, if you'd just like to collect your tickets at the desk.'

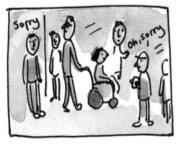

Towering desk I can't see over.
'This should be fun.'

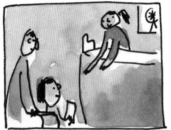

'Hello, Madam, can I take your booking reference?'
The girl stands up so she can speak to me.
I'm slightly disappointed.

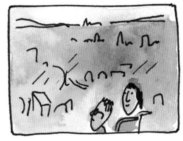

'Is everyone in? We don't want anyone rolling off!'
(Lift attendant cracks a hilarious joke.)

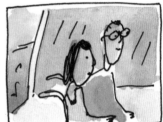

It takes half a minute to get to the 62nd floor.
Piped emotional choir music.

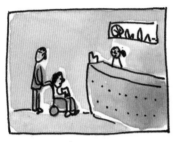

People move to let us through and say 'sorry' a lot.

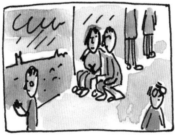

We watch lights come on across London. There's a huge black cloud with a strip of gold underneath.
'Hey look, there's the evil owl.'
(Elephant + Castle tower block.)

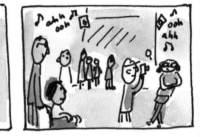

It's beautiful in every direction.
'Let's go to Crystal Palace one day.'

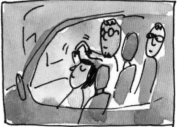

For a moment I think about dropping an atom bomb on everything and jumping off the top.

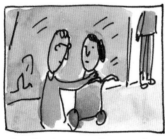

Then think about happier things.
'When shall we get married then?'
'Soon as poss?'

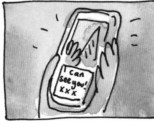

Text from Mikey.

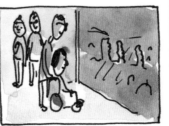

One last look at Barbican.

Mikey pulling expert U-turns on the way home.

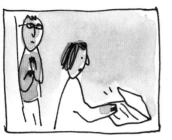

Me and Tom do lots of googling.
'Says here 6 out of 8 babies whose mothers had chemo were OK.'

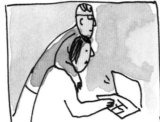

'One had a club foot, another had Asperger's.'

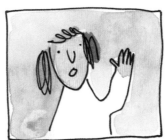

'But Asperger's ran in the family anyway.'

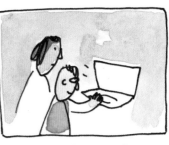

'One had a flaky patch of skin on its head.'

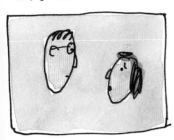

'I think we should keep the baby and start chemo now.'

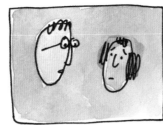

'Me too, it'll probably be alright...'
'And I really want to make sure I don't die.'

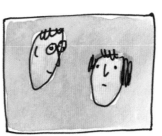

'Well, whatever happens, it'll still be nice.'

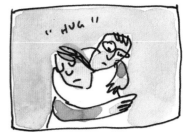

'Yeh, let's do that.'

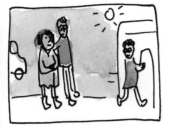

'Beautiful day!'
I can walk a short distance from the car before my stitches from the operation start hurting. Mum pops into a vintage shop.
'Just going in here!'

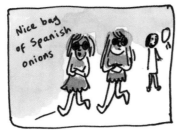

We pass two girls who look the same, talking about onions.

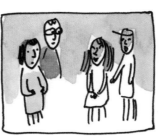

Bump into friends who've heard about the baby...
'Hey guys, amazing about the baby!'

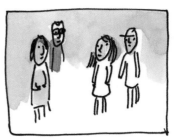

But not about the cancer. It's a bit awkward.
'Well, we're going to get some food.'

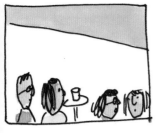

We sit outside a busy cafe next to a girl complaining about her pregnancy.

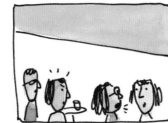

'AND I've got to cancel my holiday in Croatia because I'll be, like, eight months.'

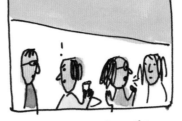

'Fuck knows how I'm going to cope with having to use a breast-feeding cushion when it's born!'

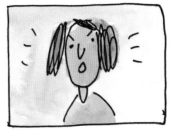

'Shall I tell her I'll have a bumbag with a chemo bottle plugged into my arm and a sock full of shit stuck to my stomach when we have ours?'
(Colostomy bag after surgery. Temporary, I hope.)

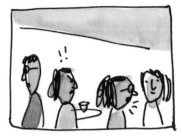

'No don't.'
'And I REALLY don't want
to give birth at my local
hospital because the
nurses are all foreign
and carry diseases.'

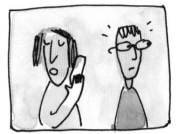

I phone my friend Adam
and enjoy talking loudly.
'Well, we had to decide
whether or not to abort
the baby before I have
chemotheraphy.'

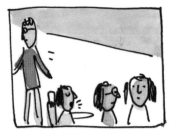

Tom goes to put more
money in the parking
meter.
'Or for me to have
chemo now and risk
damaging the baby.'

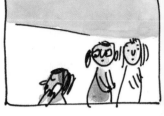

The girls look
freaked out
and leave.

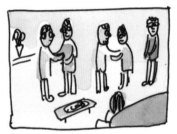

I am glad.

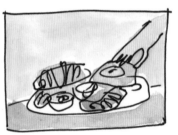

And then sad.

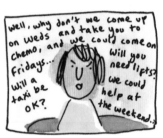

Mum's bought me a
furry snood.
'Ooh, lovely!'

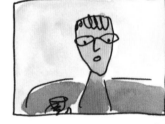

And a new coat for herself.
'I think it's rather good.'
'Me too.'

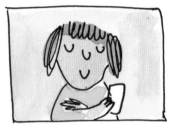

Mine and Tom's parents
meet for the first time.
'Sorry it's under such...'
(me) → 'Bad?'
'Bad, yes, bad circumstances.'

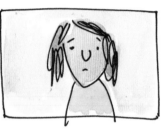

There are a LOT
of pastries.

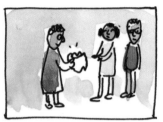

well, why don't we come up
on weds and take you to
chemo, and we could come on
Fridays... Will you
Will a need lifts?
taxi be we could
OK? help at
the weekend...

I am irritable about
planning things.
'I don't want to think
about ANY of it!'

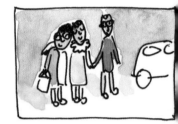

'We might go away at
the weekend before
chemo starts, maybe
to Essex.'

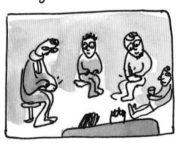

'Ooh Essex, yes Essex is lovely.'
'You could go to where Constable
is from. It's right by Suffolk.'
'Or what about Whitstable?'
(Phones all out.)

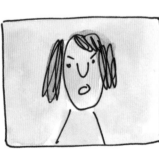

'We can find
somewhere.'

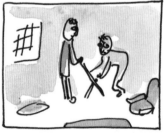

Tom and his dad
construct an exercise bike
I bought on Amazon.

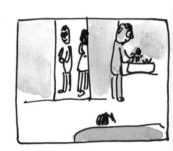

Mikey plants cyclamen
in the windowboxes and
Mum and Tom's mum
cut up avocados in the
kitchen. It's good to have
something to do.

There are a couple of harrowing things to get out of the way before the weekend.
Having my PICC line put in (a tube for chemotherapy drugs to go into).

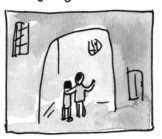

Mikey takes me to the cancer hospital. 'It's like a palace!'

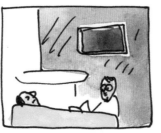

The walls in the waiting room are dark grey. 'Would you like a magazine?' 'No.'

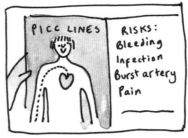

'If you could just read the form and sign.'

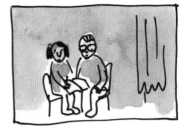

'I thought it just went into your arm.' 'Me too...'

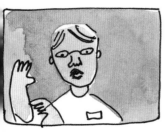

A gentle nurse explains the procedure to me using a plastic arm. 'Long, flexible wire.'

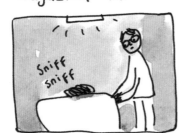

I cry before they put it in. 'Sorry.' 'Don't apologise, I'll get you some tissue. When was the diagnosis?' 'Last week.'

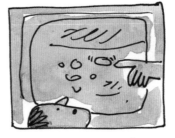

He tells me I've got nice veins and shows me an ultrasound of the inside of my arm. 'You see this? Opening and closing like a mouth? That's an artery.'

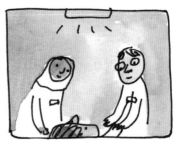

It doesn't really hurt. 'Just make a small cut here.'

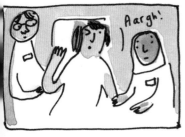

At first the line goes into my neck instead of my heart, which can happen if you've got a 'difficult anatomy'. 'Sorry, Matilda.'

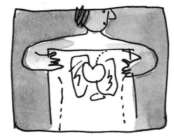

They manage to get it in my other arm. 'We just need to pull it out by 10 cm.' 'Out of where?'

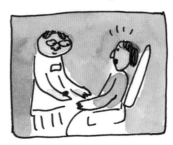

'Out of your heart.'

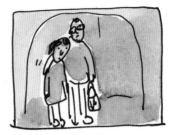

Very glad to be being looked after despite all my complaining. 'It wasn't as bad as going to the dentist.'

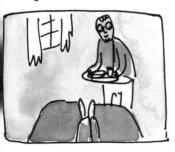

Mikey brings me consommé and grape juice... (No solids until after the endoscopy tomorrow.)

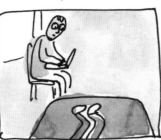

...and works on his laptop while I sleep. 'Tell me if I'm typing too loudly.'

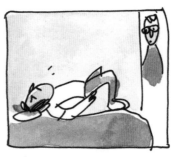

Now both arms AND my stomach are sliced up and painful, I find a new way of pushing myself up with my head. (Tom back from work.)

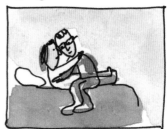

'Hi, baby, how ya doin?' 'Got the line in! It went into my neck and then into my heart.' 'Arghh! Well done.'

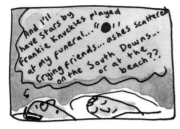

Wake up at 3 and can't get back to sleep. I try to do the imagining a dot meditation thing but my mind is racing.

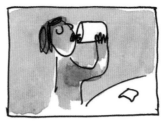

So I get up and make a start on the 4 litres of laxatives.

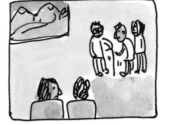

(Bowel prep for the endoscopy.)

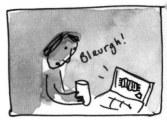

Then look at rugs and lampshades on eBay. 250ml every 15 mins for 4 hours.

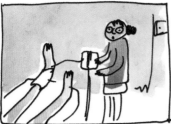

Later, a friendly 90-year-old in the waiting room wants to talk. 'More snow tonight, still, can't complain, my son lives in Sweden and it snows 6 months of the year! I went for his 60th birthday...'

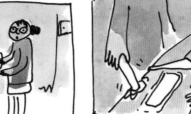

'Her son is twice my age... I shouldn't be here.'

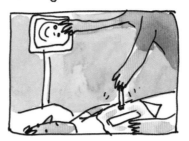

Luckily some other friendly old people step in to help with her adjustable walking stick. 'Feels like it's spring-loaded.' 'Is there a button or something?' 'Well, that just made it longer.'

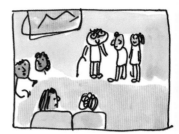

'I hope I'm like that when I'm 90.' I hope I get to BE 90. Or even 40 or 50. I feel jealous of all these oldies who've already made it.

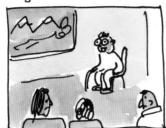

Another sweet nurse checks my blood pressure (from my leg because both arms are still messed up from the PICC line). 'And pregnant as well?' I enjoy telling her all about it.

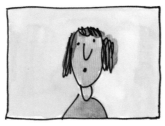

Camera on a stick poked into the new hole in my side. I must've been invented by David Cronenberg. (It's not actually as bad as it looks.)

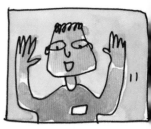

'Polyps at 12, 6 and 9 o'clock.' They take some biopsies just in case, but don't seem that worried.

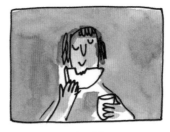

'If worst came to worst we could take out your whole bowel!'

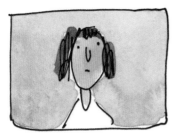

'Ah, good.'

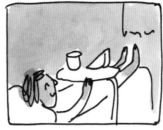

I feel like Noomi Rapace in Prometheus, except I get a cup of tea and a cheese sandwich instead of an aborted squid alien.

Nicest thing I ever ate.

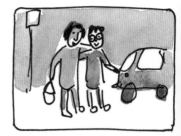

'Nothing looked malignant.' 'Phew!' 'And I got a free pair of arseless shorts.' 'Haha!'

Tom and me spend the weekend in Mersea (Essex) before chemo starts. Freezing and beautiful.

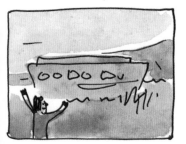

'Decay!'
We look at a lot of rotten boats.

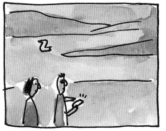

'I think that's the North Kent coast.'
'No it isn't, we're looking West, that's an estuary. See?'

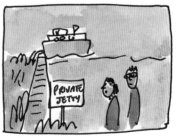

'Don't worry, we didn't want to touch your silly old boat anyway.'
(Did quite want to.)

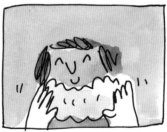

Grateful for my furry snood.

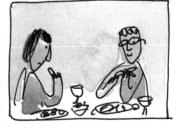

Huge seafood platter. Think about how many creatures I'm eating. Elderflower cordial instead of wine.

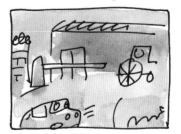

We try to find a Roman barrow and end up in an industrial estate.
'I swear this road said it went somewhere.'

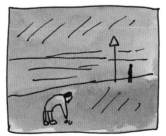

Pick up oyster shells on the beach in the gloaming.

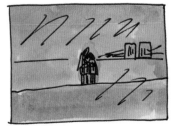

No wind at all. We look across the water at Bradwell nuclear power station (decommissioned 2002).

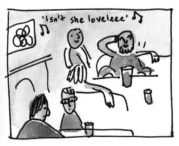

'Isn't she loveleee'
Heavy thoughts in cheery pub about why I got cancer and this guy didn't.
'If she came in here I'd kick her on the floor and stick a candle in her eye.'

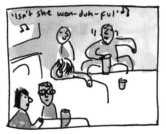

'Isn't she won-duh-ful'
'Don't know if I can stay for pudding, those people are darking me out.'
'I was like why the fuck did you indicate then not pull out?! Stupid fucker. Got his glasses and chucked them over a wall.'

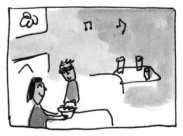

They leave and I have rice pudding with jam and cream.
'There's room for a bit more rice pudding under your chin.'

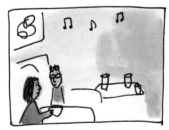

Talk a little bit about how we're feeling.
'Thing is, we can't really go back to normal, and I don't like being looked after.'
'Better let them take you to chemo a few times.'

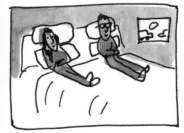

Back at the B+B, I talk to Jim on the phone. He sounds more shaken up than me.
'Oh my God. I just want to give you a hug! Fucking hell. That's really knocked me for six.'
'Well, I know, but there might not even be any cells left.'

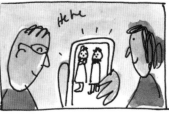

He sends me a photo of him and his dad looking exactly the same to cheer me up.

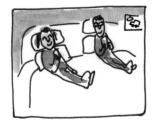

We both contentedly go on our phones, with Jeremy Clarkson playing rugby in cars with a giant ball on TV in the background.

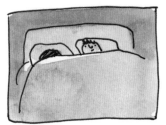

That night I feel the baby kick for the first time.
'Give me your hand... feel that? That?'
'I think so...'

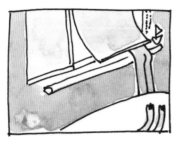

In the morning;
'Ah yes, grey sky, grey sea.'

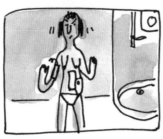

Forget to bring cling film to waterproof my bandages and can't use the power shower. 'Damn!'

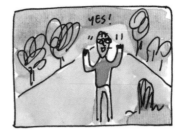

On the way home, we finally find the Roman barrow next to a barn conversion and a chicken shed.

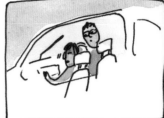

It's sometimes hard for Tom to tell if I'm laughing or crying. Laughing this time, lot of mileage in those arseless shorts.

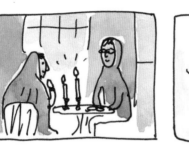

Heating's been off all weekend at the flat so we keep our coats on and eat crumpets by candle light.

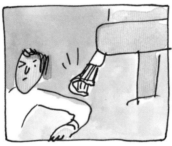

Tom's mum's gerberas are still doing well after three weeks.

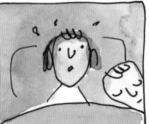

I go on the exercise bike and watch Waltz with Bashir on MUBI.

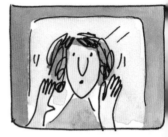

Just managed to grow my hair long enough to flick around. Worry about it all falling out.

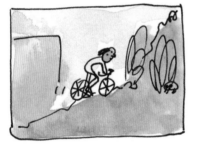

I have terrible dreams about escaping from hospital on a broken bike.

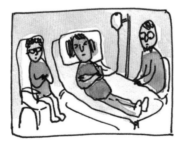

And being identity marked by a horse's hoof in a pneumatic stamping machine.

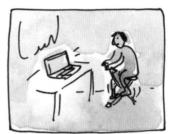

Wake up in a cold sweat several nights in a row.

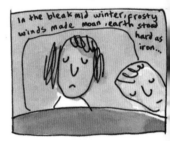

Recalling the words to Christmas carols calms me down, slightly.

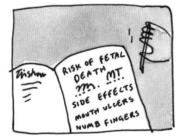

First dose of chemotherapy. My initials look cheerful next to 'Risk of fetal death'.

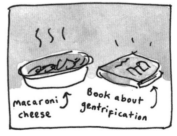

Terrified I'm going to miscarry or die of a toxic reaction.

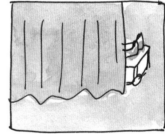

But it's mostly uneventful.

Apart from an argument I have with the woman next door about whether to have the curtain open or closed. 'She's had it closed all day! It's so dark in here!' 'I want some privacy!'

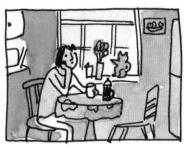

Things settle down a bit and there's time to reflect between fortnightly doses of chemo.

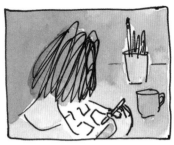

It helps to draw it all.

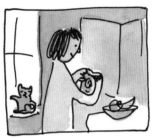

The pregnancy had been quite easy so far. I was eating a lot of pickled onion crisps.

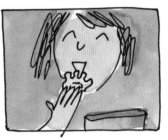

But I do that anyway!

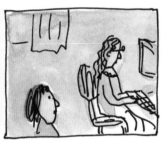

I had been to the doctor about a sharp pain in my stomach. 'It comes and goes...'

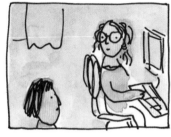

'... and sometimes my shit looks like jam.'

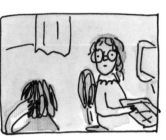

'But, um, I've had piles before so maybe it's that.'

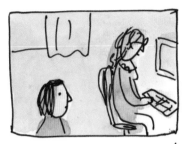

'Try taking some Gaviscon.' It was probably pregnancy symptoms.

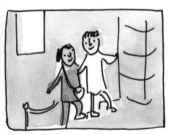

I went to meet Adam at the Royal Academy for the Mariko Mori exhibition. 'Any pregnancy symptoms?' 'Not really, bit bloated but that's about it.'

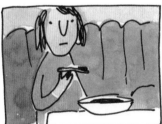

I had just tried to eat some tomato soup at Patisserie Valerie on Piccadilly...

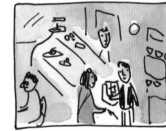

They were sweet about not making me pay. 'She can't eat it, she's pregnant.' 'That's fine, Madam, have a lovely day.'

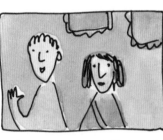

Me and Adam talk about our friends. 'He cancelled to go and pick his boyfriend up from the station again!' 'What?! The guy's been to London before, right?'

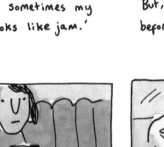

'Wait... I've got to go and be sick right now.'

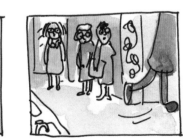

Run to the loo past a lot of old ladies. 'There's a queue!'

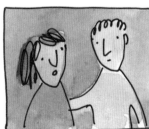

'Think I'd better go, just projectiled.'

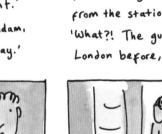

Adam gets some carrier bags in case I'm sick on the way home. 'Small or big?' 'Um, big. More please. Thanks.' We didn't see the show.

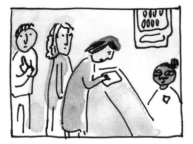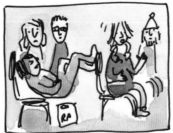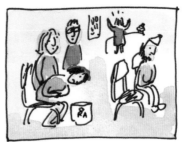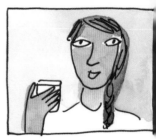

Later that night, Claire takes me to A+E.
'13 weeks pregnant, can't stop being sick, in loads of pain...'
'Take a seat please.'

We wait for ages.
Tom comes after work.
A girl gets annoyed about losing a pound in the vending machine.
'I'm sorry but it's not good enough.'

'You're definitely more ill than her.'
'Someone is responsible for this!'

They've run out of specimen pots so a doctor gives me a plastic cup to pee in.

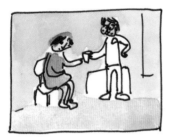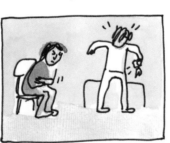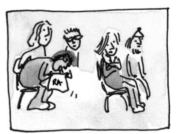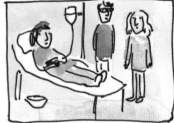

I give it to a nurse.
'Wait, what's this?'

Who spills it down her trousers.
'This is outrageous! who told you to pee in here?'
'I can't remember, they ran out of wee pots.'

We wait another hour while she changes her clothes.
'Silly woman. You'd think she'd be used to getting a bit of wee on her trousers.'

I'm given a drip and some painkillers.
'You be alright if I go?'
'Yeh.'

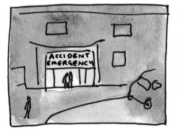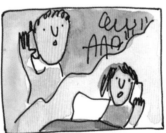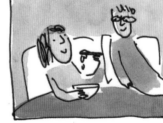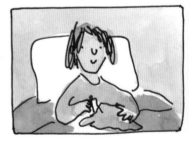

And sent home.
'Let's get a taxi.'

Speak to Adam.
'Did you get back OK?'
'Just, had to go to A+E. They said I've got norovirus, really hope you don't get it!'

Tom makes me some watery soup.
'Delicious!'

And I darn jumpers.

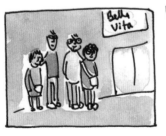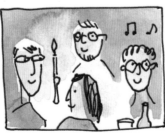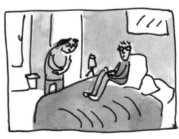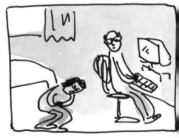

My parents come up and we go for some supper.
'I could probably manage some fish...'

'What is this familiar music?'
'Michael Jackson.'
'I think Tom could manage some pudding.'

I'm still getting stomach pain two weeks later.
'Better go back to the doctor.'
'Will you come with me?'
'Yeh course.'

See a different GP.
'Can't you give me some anti-cramping medicine? Gaviscon didn't help.'
'Hmm, I think it'd be wise to go back to A+E. I'll write you a letter.'

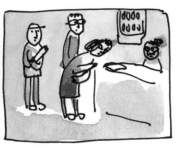

'15 weeks pregnant, can't stop being sick, really bad stomach pain...'
'Take a seat please.'

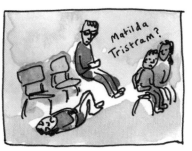

It's less painful to lie on the floor. Tom tells work he can't make it.

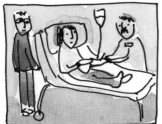

Given a drip, painkillers and anti-sickness medicine.
'And I haven't done a shit for a week. Is that important?'

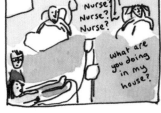

Taken to a busy ward.

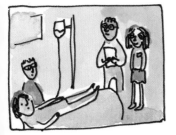

No one seems to know what to do with me.
'Are you in pain? Are you vomiting?'
'Not as much but I've had painkillers and anti-sickness medicine.'

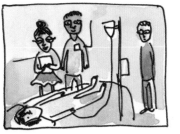

Lots of trendy young doctors come and go.
'What we're going to do is we're going to scan the baby, make sure that's all OK.'

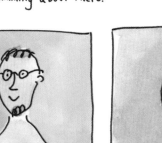

'Mm, you've got a brick wall of gas in your intestines and a bit of free fluid. But the baby's looking fine, lovely, swimming about there.'

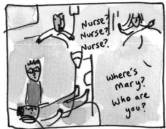

Back to the busy ward.

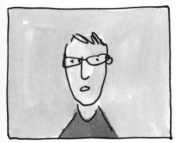

It's Friday and all the young doctors are going home for the weekend.
'But what about the fluid and brick wall of gas?'

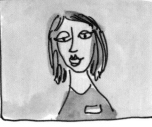

'Pregnancy can cause digestive problems. Try eating something if you can.'

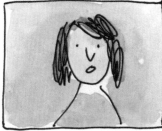

'If I were you I'd go home, it's mayhem in here at the weekend, and come back on Monday if you're still in pain.'

Tom/img — 'I'm not going home again, it's obviously getting worse!'

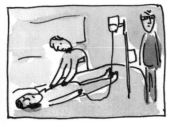

'What if there's a blockage? Isn't there another scan she can have?'

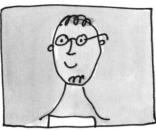

'You'll have to talk to my colleague on Monday, I won't be here because I'm going on holiday to Morocco in the morning.'

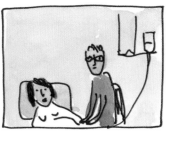

'Oh, lucky you. I hope you don't get anything gastro.'

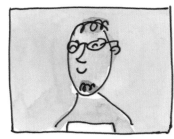

'Thanks!'

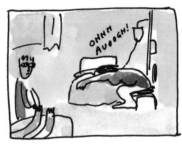

It's a long weekend.
A woman opposite's gastric band has gone wrong.

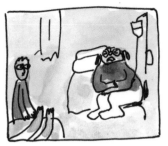

'This really isn't good enough, I've been here since TUESDAY!'
(Poor woman.)

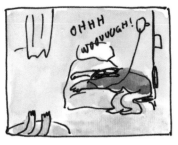

She howls all night like a wounded dog.

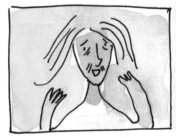

Another lady thinks we're all at a party.
'Did Mary organise this?'
'Shh, dear, you've broken your pelvis, go to sleep.'
'Who are you?' etc.

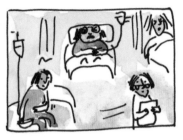

There aren't many doctors around and we all compete for attention.
'Please! I feel like I'm going to explode!'
'OHHH!'
'Tell Mary to take me home!!'

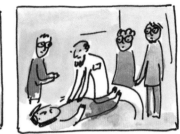

Tom and my parents arrive.
'They let 3 of us in.'
Mikey googles 'gastric obstruction'.
'Can be detected with an MRI scan.'

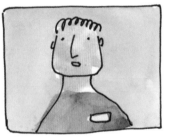

The doctors aren't convinced.
'Feels like trapped wind.'
'Can't you give her an MRI just to rule it out?'

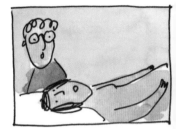

'We could go and get it done privately!'
'Shh, don't say that!'
(Luckily he'd already gone.)

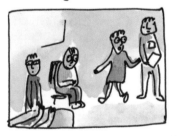

Mum runs off down the ward and grabs another doctor.
'Please, it's urgent, my daughter's pregnant and in terrible pain!'
'I'm not even supposed to be working here today.'

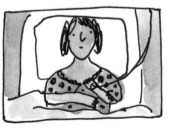

Examined again.
'Well, you're right, it could be an obstruction.'

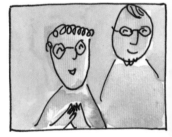

'I will request an MRI.'

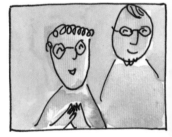

'Oh, thank you so much!! At last.'

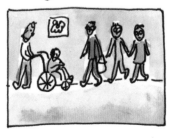

Am taken to another ward.
(They wheel you backwards.)

Given a flowery nightie.
'Bit hetero-normative, isn't it.'

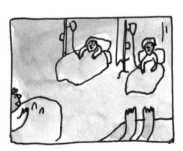

The women on my ward are very chatty.
'My friend Ros, her husband is an IT technician, she had a dog once, like a daughter she was...'

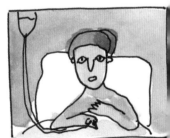

And quite deaf.
'Shih Tzu. Shih Tzu! It was a SHIH TZU, Iris!'
I pretend to be asleep.

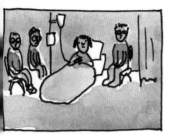

Monday morning, expecting an MRI scan.

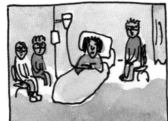

Nothing happens for hours. 'I don't believe this...'

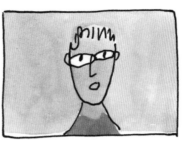

'What's happening about this MRI scan? They said they'd do it today, we've been here since Thursday and no one's doing anything!'

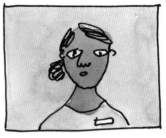

'I'll ask the doctor to come.'

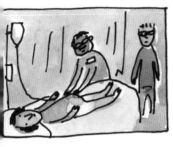

Another doctor comes. 'If you had an abortion we could give you an X-Ray to see what's going on.'

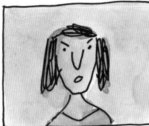

'I don't want an abortion!'

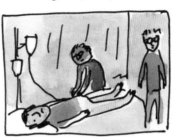

And another doctor. 'Does it hurt here?' 'It hurts everywhere!' 'Could be appendicitis, I'll prescribe some antibiotics in case that helps.'

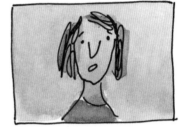

'WHAT?!'

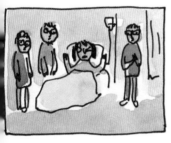

'Antibiotics? Are they completely insane? What if it's a blockage and my insides rupture?!'

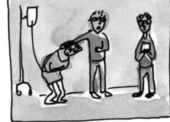

We plead with a nervous young doctor. 'Yesterday they said they'd scan her, we NEED to make sure it's not an obstruction, she could die if it is!'

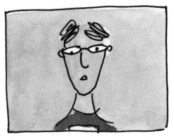

'The problem is that the MRI machines aren't owned or managed by the NHS... we need two doctors' signatures and their consent, there are waiting lists...'

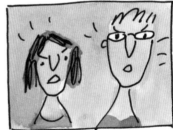

FURY

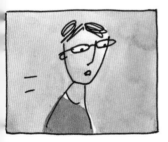

'I'll see what I can do.' He seemed to sympathise.

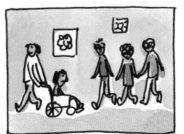

They arrange another ultrasound scan instead.

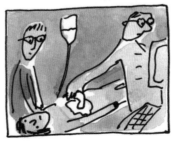

The radiographer takes a long time over it.

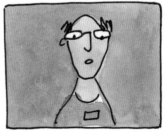

'She needs an MRI scan. I'll see if they can fit you in now.'

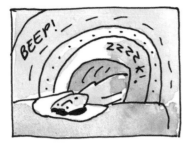

They fit me in straight away.
'Breathe in please, Matilda.'
The machine sounds like
breakcore. I think about
DJ Scotch Egg and raves
at the Electrowerks.

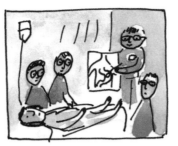

Back at the ward, a friendly
surgeon comes to see us.
'There is a total blockaage
in your sigmoid colon and
we're going to operate
first thing tomorrow.'

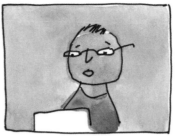

'I'd do it tonight but I
want the team to be fresh.
Looks like a tumour of
some sort, probably benign,
but we'll remove a foot
of your large bowel and
test it just in case.'

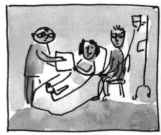

My intestines are so
stretched they have to do
open surgery instead of
laparoscopic (keyhole).
'We'll do everything we can
to protect your baby.
Sign here, please.'

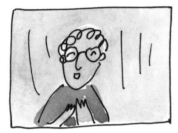

'At last, I could kiss him!'

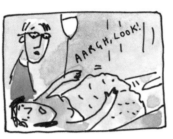

That night, you can see
the outline of my intestines
straining under my skin.

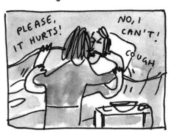

Another doctor tries to
put a tube up my nose and
down my throat to relieve
some of the pressure.
I am sick on her hands.

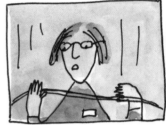

'You have to.
Come on, be brave.'

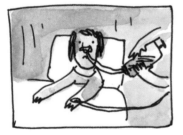

Eventually she gets it in
and sucks out 2 pints
of dark green bile.
Just like pond water.
It helps a bit.

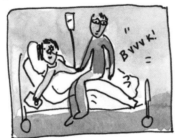

The nurses let Tom stay
till 10. Distract ourselves
with the adjustable bed.
'Just like sitting on a
grassy hillock.'

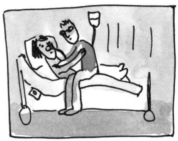

'I'm scared.'
'You're wonderful.'
'I wish you could stay
till tomorrow...'
'Me too!'

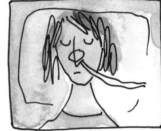

I listen to a Melvyn Bragg
podcast about Pitt Rivers
and try to sleep.

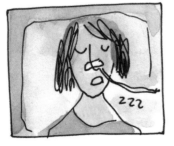

The one about Norse gods
does the trick.

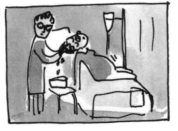

Mum is allowed in early
to wash my hair before
the operation.

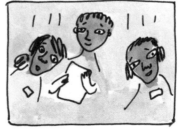

The nurses are all praying
for me and the baby.
'God will look after you,
my dear.'

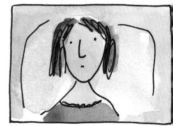

Not sure about that.

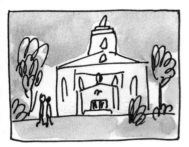

Tom and Mikey walk around Hackney while the doctors operate. (St John's church.)

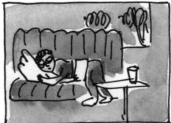

Mum does the cryptic crossword in the restaurant by the ward and falls asleep.

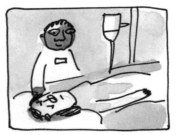

'Wake up, darling... Wake up, dear... You're OK, the operation went fine. My name is Veronica and I'll be looking after you today.'

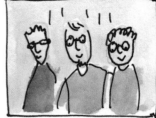

Tom, Mum and Mikey are allowed in, briefly. 'Well done, darling.'

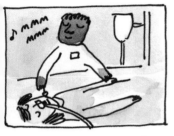

My heart rate won't go down so I'm kept in observation until the evening. Veronica hums songs from Les Mis and dabs my mouth with a wet sponge. It's very comforting.

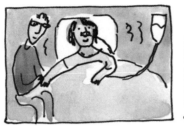

Back on the ward, painkillers are great. 'I'm radiating clouds of love for you...' (Tom said it was like being in a chill-out room, but it's true, I was radiating clouds of love!)

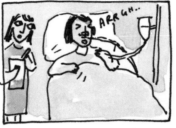

Until they wear off. 'How bad is it on a scale of 1 to 10, 1 being fine, 10 being unbearable?' 'Unbearable! 10!' It really hurt.

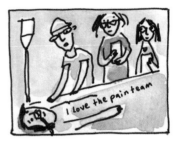

'We've given you morphine for now, you can have top-ups of oxycontin if you need it.' The pain team sorted me out.

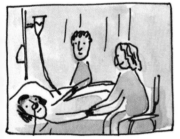

Claire and Adam visit. 'I've got to have a colostomy bag for about a year.' 'Argh!' 'But at least I'm alive.'

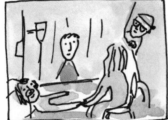

The anaesthetist comes to check I'm OK. I like the familiar way he calls us 'guys'. 'Fine, thanks, can't feel a thing.'

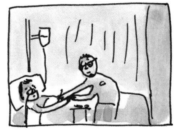

Holiday-in-Morocco Doc comes to do blood tests, he looks sheepish. 'It's lucky we didn't send you home, isn't it?' (Lucky I refused to go, more like.)

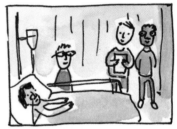

Two more trendy doctors come to ask if I want a hot-water bottle. They seem like good friends, in matching Converse and skinny jeans. 'Got this hot bag of shit warming me up so I don't think I'll need one, thanks.'

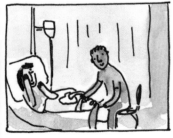

In the morning, one of them comes to listen for the baby's heart (still beating) and I cry. 'Amazing.' 'Ah there, you see? It is tough. Probably a lovely little girl.'

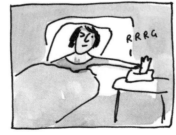

By now, I can just about move to reach a tissue.

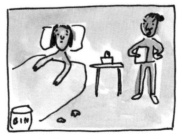

Am told off by the ward manager for dropping them on the floor. 'Don't expect us to do everything for you, put them in the bin!' There's an inspection.

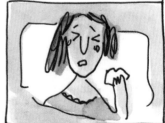

'I can't reach the bin! It's a triumph I can even reach the tissues!' Boo hoo hoo etc.

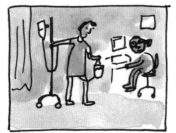

A few days later, I can walk to the bathroom ('mobilising').
'Look at you on the catwalk!'
A girl can never have too many accessories.

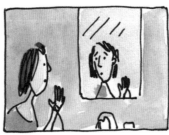

I am shocked by how thin I am. Big eyelids.

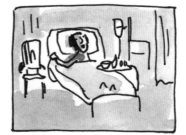

Explain to a new patient how to use the emergency button and feel like a veteran.
'Just press this thing that looks like a bullet and the nurses come.'

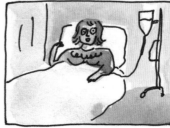

She talks a lot about house prices in Stoke Newington and I miss the lady with the shih tzu.
'There are a lot of Hasidic Jewish people at my doctor's surgery and they're all lovely.'

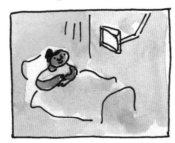

Another new woman in the bed next door is about to have a gastric band fitted.
'I'm not even allowed milkshakes or ice cream.'

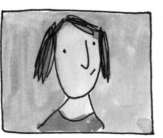

Feel like warning her after seeing the other gastric band lady.

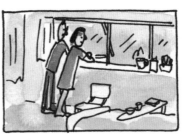

Have the catheter taken out. It's good to stand up and look out of the open window.

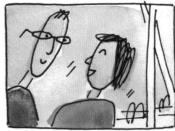

'What a relief, that thing was really taking the piss!'
'Ha!'

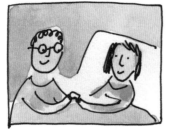

Mum brings me a replica Vogelherd mammoth from the Ice Age exhibition at the British Museum.

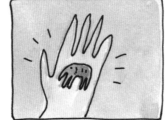

'Imagine, 35,000 years. I love it!'

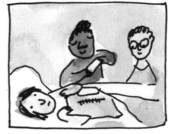

A nurse changes my bandage and I notice that I haven't got a belly button any more.
Mum thinks she can still see it.
'A mother's eye...'

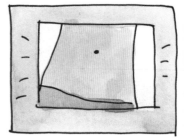

I'm sad I didn't take a photo of it, or something. It was a nice belly button.

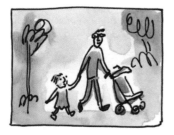

The little girl Tom looks after knows there's something going on.
'Matty's OK, isn't she?'
'Yes, she is, she's being looked after by good doctors.'

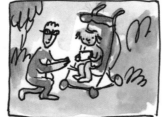

'Hmm... But what if there are trees in my kangaroo sandwich??'

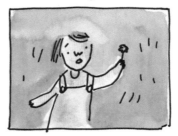

Sometimes she has French New Wave days.
'Flowers are pretty, but I don't like flowers because they die.'

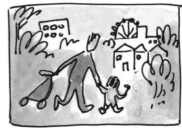

'Everything dies apart from houses.'

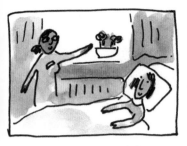

One nurse takes a liking to the miniature roses from my dad.
'So pretty!'

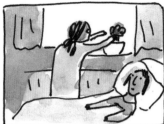

'Yes, they're not very happy with the heaters on so high.' She takes the dead bits off.

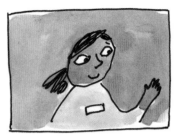

'I could take them? Bit better outside!'

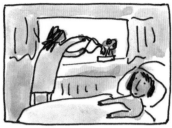

'Well, yes, I mean, let's wait and see how they're doing later on.'

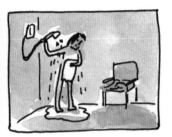

I manage to have a shower, holding a towel over the stitches etc.

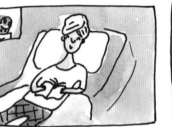

Put on my own clothes, feeling good about going home the next day.

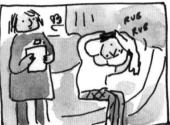

A different nurse comes to talk to me.
'And how are you feeling about the diagnosis tomorrow?'
'Well, er, I don't think there's much point worrying.'

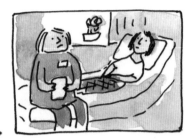

'Mm, and how are you feeling about the difficult decisions you might have to make?'
'It's probably benign so I might not have to make them.'

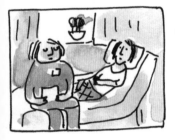

'Obviously, if I do have to make them it will be awful.'
'Mmm.'

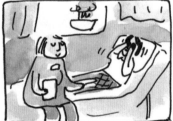

(CRIES)
'Yes, and we're here to help you through that.'

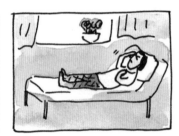

I was feeling fine before she came!

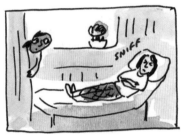

'Oh! You're crying...'

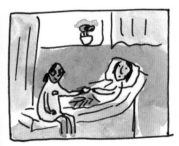

'Don't cry, here, have a tissue. Tough cookie you are. How are the flowers?'
'Oh, still a bit dry.'

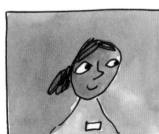

'I take them?'

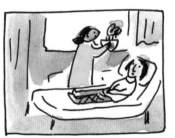

'Yes, why not, they'll be happier.'

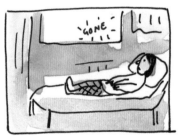

I feel a bit bereft.

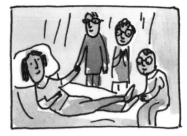 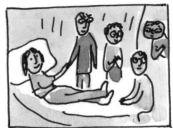 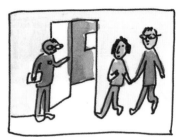 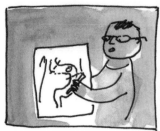

My parents and Tom come to collect me the next morning. 'Darling, you look so much better!'

The surgeon arrives. 'Matilda, everyone, if you'd like to follow me...'

A tiny, windowless room. I try not to think: 'It must be bad news.'

'The bad news is that I'm afraid the tumour was cancerous.'

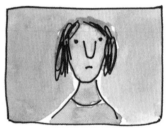 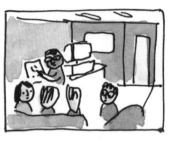 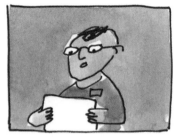 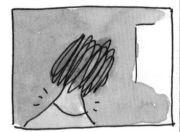

I don't feel anything.

'The good news is that of the 25 lymph nodes we removed, only 5 were infected.'

'So we'll give you a course of mild chemotherapy to mop up any leftover cells.'

I am surprised to notice that the only reaction to being told I've got a potentially terminal disease is that my neck feels suddenly icy cold.

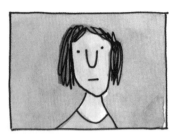 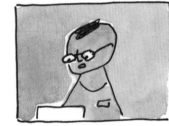 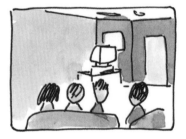 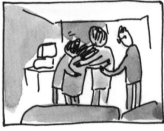

I think, 'This is the moment we hug each other and cry.'

'I'll let you have some space for a bit.'

We hug each other and cry.

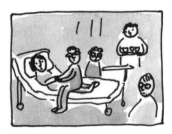 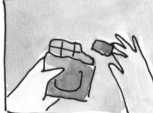 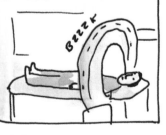 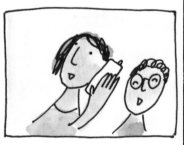

We're quickly moved to a private room off the ward and brought cups of sweet tea.

Mum's got some Ritter Sport.

I have a CT scan to see if it's spread to my liver or lungs.

It hasn't.

MARCH

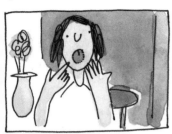

I have a few weird side effects after the first dose of chemo.
'Tongue feels like a scotch egg.' But nothing major.

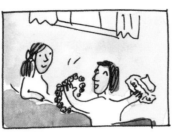

Cesca comes with presents from India: a plastic flower garland and a baroque tissue box.
'Haha, brilliant, I have become a tissue person!'

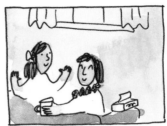

'This naked woman massaged my head while Ed bought an electronic raga machine.'
'Coool.' Enjoy not talking about cancer.

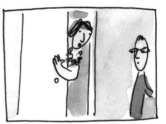

Later that night...
'Help! My shit looks like cappuccino!'

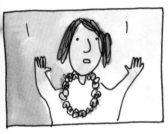

'Both parts, the froth and the coffee!'

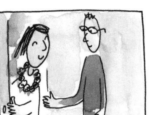

'What about the powdered heart?'
'Hehe, no.'

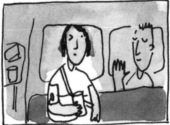

Sleeping with the chemo pump attached is quite annoying. It's a little bottle of drugs that goes into my arm over 2 days, once a fortnight.

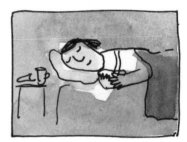

I pretend I'm sleeping at an airport and it's a money belt I really don't want to get stolen. It works quite well.

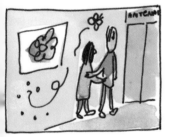

The following week Tom and me go for the 20-week scan.

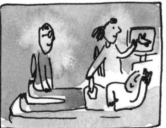

Cry again when it's all OK. 'All these measurements are looking good, he's growing fine, placentas are amazing things.'

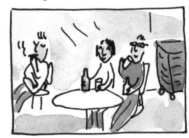

Relieved apple juice in the sun next to a wheelie bin on Chatsworth Road.
Fun thinking of silly names.
'Mork? Imhotep?'

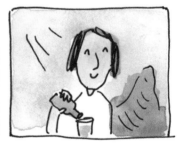

'Gandalf?'

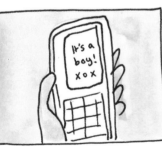

Tell my aunts they can start tentatively knitting again.

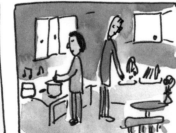

Will have lots of check-ups to make sure chemo isn't damaging my placenta.
'We can make a toxic risotto out of it, haha.'

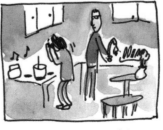

Hearing music I like suddenly makes me cry harder than I've ever known. It's like sneezing or being sick.

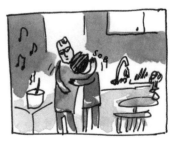

Feel like if I don't cling on to Tom I'll sink into the floor.

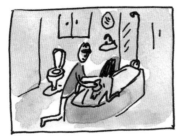

Tom washes my back in the bath (got to keep chemo arm out of the water).

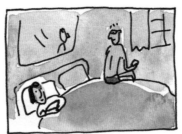

'You setting an alarm for tomorrow?'
'Yeh, 8 o'clock.'
I want to hear his alarm go off in the morning thousands more times.

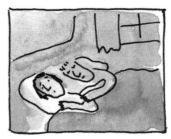

Panic to think that I might not.

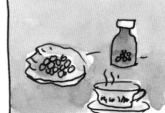

Remembering things from my grandparents' house stops me from thinking about dying any time soon. Marbles in a shell, smell of lapsang souchong, pink ibuprofen pills.

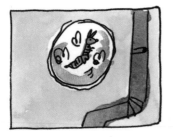

Plate on the wall above the Aga with a picture that looked like a rabbit with its bum showing (the bum was actually part of the rabbit's bicep).

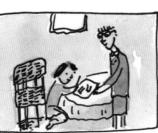

Trying to draw horses' hooves in the conservatory, aged about 5, Nan showing me how.

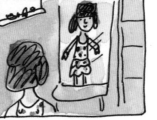

The way their wicker chair felt on my knees when the cushion had gone astray.

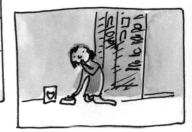

By their dark larder seeing what cat biscuits taste like (also aged 5).

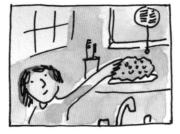

Feeling a natural sponge in their bathroom.

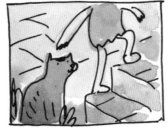

Clay cat outside the back door that had a hole in the top of its head.

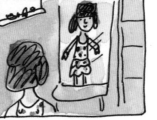

Looking at myself in the hall mirror in a too big Russian hat.

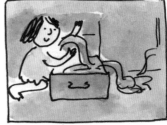

The smell of Nan's drawer full of scarves from trips round the world (perfume and polish).

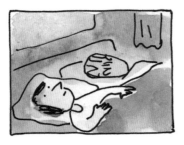

I often wake up with 'moderately differentiated adinocarcinoma' or similar, going round in my mind.

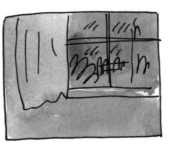

Guess what time it is by how many cars are going by outside. Not many. About 4.30.

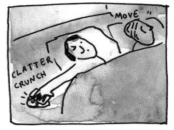

Go on my phone for a bit and accidentally put it down loudly in a plate of crystals my sister sent.

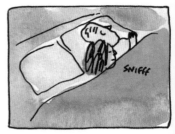

Inhaling Tom's shoulder is comforting.

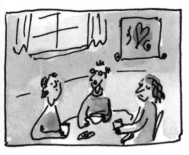

Hannah has difficult conversations with hippie friends.
'Chemo's more likely to kill her than cancer, you know.'

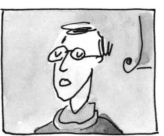

'She ought to be treated homoeopathically.'

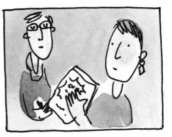

They give her a book that recommends cutting out 'corpse sugar', having psychotherapy and taking psyllium husk.

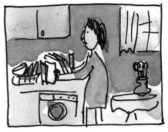

I hide it between cookery books with its spine facing inwards.

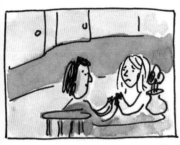

Amy comes to see me and cries.
'I can't believe you're having to go through this!'
'I know, it's shit.'

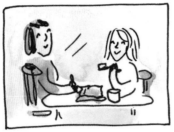

We go to a cafe, share a big apple cake and talk about a sitcom she's writing (and lots of other stuff).
'We're having to think less like actors, more like writers.'

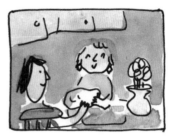

Michelle brings me a giant meringue from Dulwich.
'You'd better eat like a sumo wrestler now!'
'Cor, thanks!'

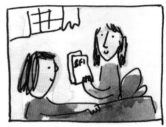

Pia brings some DVDs and cooks me pasta.
We talk about animations we plan to make.
'What do you think about strata-cutting?'
'Everywhere at the moment.'

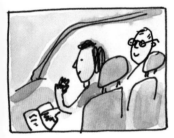

My cousin, Alex, drives me to get my PICC line dressing changed. Eat rice crispy cakes and look at Duckman comic in the car.

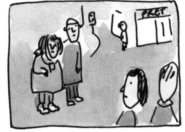

Starting to recognise people on their way to hospital.
Tired-looking, too many clothes, stiff wigs. Would never have noticed them before.

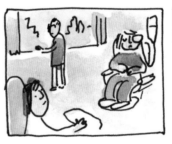

On the ward there's a woman with a chemo drip going straight into her eye.
Alex looks out of the window. There's a great view.

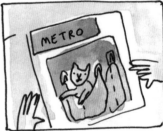

There are soothing stories in the Metro about cats climbing into suitcases.

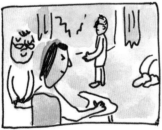

I still feel squeamish about looking at the PICC line.
The nurse can tell and asks where I live.
'Oh, Hackney Road, I live near there too!'

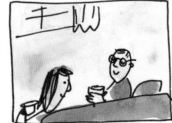

Back at home, Alex is wise about colostomy bags.
'Imagine if everyone had one and the doctors told you, "sorry, we're going to move your arsehole really far up a hairy crack that's hard to reach" you'd think it was terrible!'

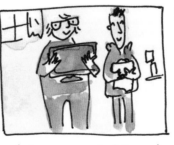

Later, my aunt Polly and cousin Felix bring round a TV and a Wii.
'Sorry about the bag of SCART leads.'

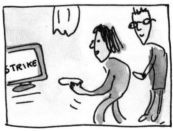

I enjoy bowling more than I am expecting to.
'Yesss!'

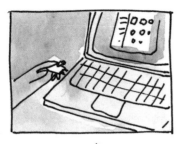

I transfer a file of one of my films to send to a man at the British Film Council. It's the first normal thing I've done for ages.

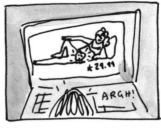

Fuzzbutt wants to chat!

Then join a colostomy forum. They're all about 70 and seem to enjoy a 'healthy sex life'.

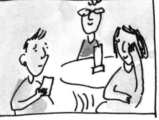

★29.99

ARGH!

I freak myself out looking at lacy colostomy bag covers.

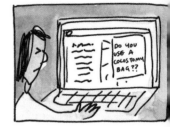

Do you use a colostomy bag??

Now all the ads that appear when I use Google are for colostomy products. I can never use my laptop for teaching again!

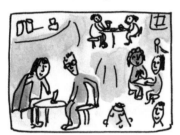

Me and Tom go to the Market Cafe to meet Matt.
'I think we'll all fit in here.'

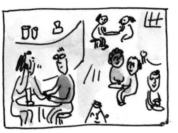

Seeing people enjoying breakfast together and not having to deal with cancer makes me cry.

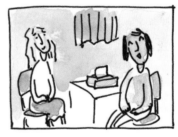

A concerned waiter kneels down to take our order.
'Just a peppermint tea please.'
'And a cappuccino.'

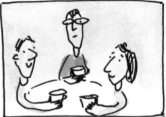

I cheer up just in time before Matt arrives. We talk about juicers...
'Aren't they hard to clean?'
And documentaries about steam power.
'I can't remember how it worked.'

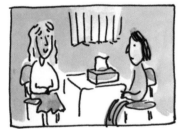

I go to see a crisis counsellor (suggested by my GP). There's a HUGE box of tissues on the table.

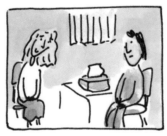

I've never had counselling before and am surprised that she doesn't say very much and it's up to me to decide what to talk about.
'So, er, I don't know how I'm going to stop worrying about dying and stuff...'

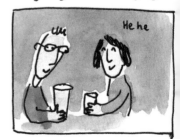

'And I can't believe I've got to deal with all this shit when I should be sitting on a lotus leaf relaxing before I have a baby.'

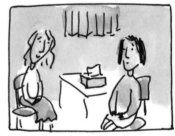

She notices I keep laughing when I'm describing it all and wonders how I feel about that. 'Um, I dunno really. I guess if I wasn't laughing I'd be crying.'

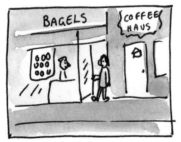

BAGELS   COFFEE HAUS

She said I seemed to be dealing with it well and perhaps I didn't need counselling. Walk to the bagel shop on Brick Lane (the furthest I've walked for ages) and buy two with cream cheese and gherkin.

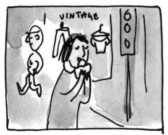

VINTAGE

Eat them both on the way home. The best therapy.

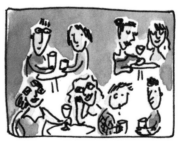

Later, me and Tom go to the pub round the corner. It's reassuring to see everything carrying on as normal. Gorgeous girls and boys in tweed calling each other 'old bean'.
'All these girls make me feel so unsexy! Trampy old clothes, haven't washed for days...'

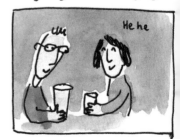

He he

'But you always wear those clothes.'
'Oh yeah.'

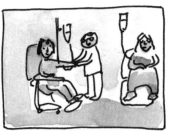

Go for a second dose of chemo and wonder if I'm being too cheerful. 'Hi there! How are you? No tea thanks.'

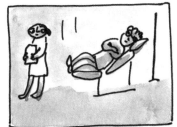

Mum falls asleep in one of the treatment chairs.

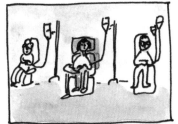

Everyone else is old. They seem to look at me with a mixture of sympathy and relief that at least they're not as young as me. We are just far apart enough not to have to talk to each other.

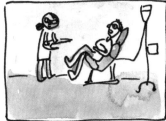

One old guy in expensive-looking shoes tells the nurse all about how he just gave each of his sisters £1000.

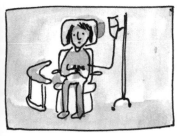

I'm glad to have the baby as an extra companion in the chemo room, a new life to think about instead of death.

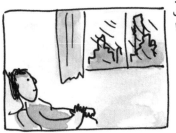

The slipped jet stream is making the weather terrible all the time. I don't mind, it makes me resent being in hospital less.

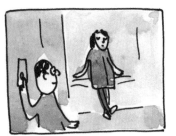

In the lift on the way down. 'You look very regally pregnant, darling.' 'Thanks, Mum.'

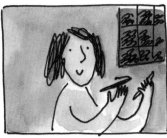

There's a great pen shop on the way home.

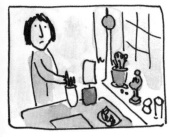

Add new pens to the pot on my desk and wonder what Tom would do with all my things if I died.

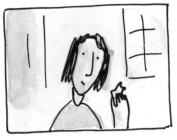

It's really hard not to think about stuff like that.

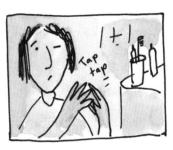

Not many bad symptoms this time either. Slightly numb fingers as if I've been playing the ukulele for hours, but not much else.

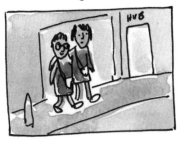

Me and Mum go to the shops to celebrate chemo not being too bad. I want to find a coat that isn't black so I don't feel like I'm going to my own funeral the whole time.

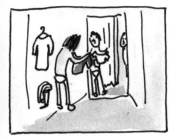

Try on a lot of stuff while Mum strokes handbags. The curtain isn't quite closed and I notice the shop guy noticing my colostomy bag.

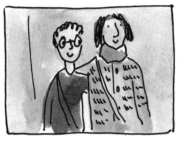

Find a green and blue coat with woven stripes. 'Just like rain on a spring day.' 'It can be my birthday present.'

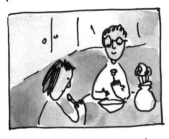

Mum makes a fish and lentil stew. Very good.

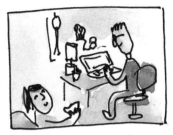

Tom gets back and we play songs on YouTube and eat cheese on toast. 'I love this one. What is it again?' Just like old times.

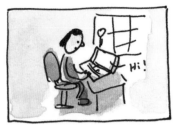

I've arranged to be part of a Skype book club.
'Hello!'

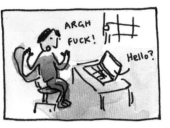

Colostomy bag suddenly leaks everywhere. Luckily, we had video turned off.

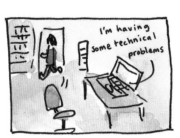

I pretend to have to take a phonecall.
'Back in 15 mins!'

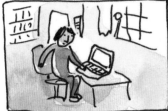

'Hello? Can you hear me?' We decide to meet in real life instead.

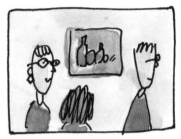

Tom's Mum, Tom and me go to the Morandi exhibition at the Estorick Collection.
'Just Fabulous!'

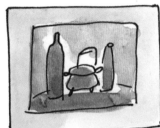

Lots of calm bottles.

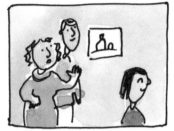

I enjoy eavesdropping.
'It's just nothing new to me, you know?'

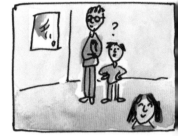

And in the permanent collection.
'How is THAT about dance?'

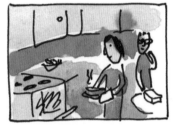

It's my birthday at the weekend, I bake two cakes, one made of black beans.
'Mmm, smells delicious.'
'Looks like a cowpat.'

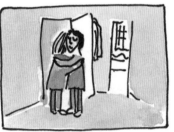

Have a few friends over. We laugh about things and I realise I haven't thought about cancer for maybe an hour.
'Maths is stupid.'
'Haha.'

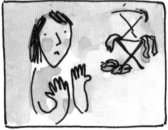

Everyone's gone by 7o'clock.
'Bye dude, love you.'
Last year we all gatecrashed a party full of people with their faces painted blue who gave us absinthe and had bad paintings of mushrooms on their walls.

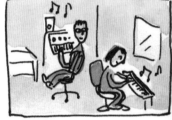

Later, me and Tom play on our new synth arrangement.
'Haha, sounds shit, doesn't it?'
'Yep.'

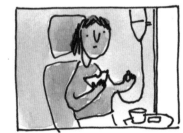

Have another chemo dose before going to my parents' in Sussex for my _actual_ birthday. Have a cheese and onion sandwich and loads of steroids.

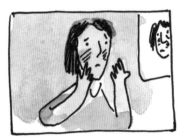

The steroids make my face go purple.

My hands go red and swell up. Can't hang up the washing. Feels like chilblains.

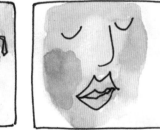

Swollen lips look quite good though.

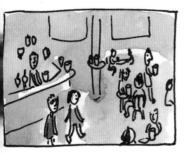

Stop at a Wetherspoon's in Norbury on the way to Sussex so I can go to the loo.
'Look at all these people, boozing away, not having cancer...'

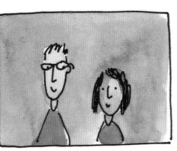

'Ah it's OK, some of them probably do.'

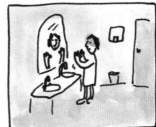

Wash my weird red hands very carefully and look at them in the mirror.

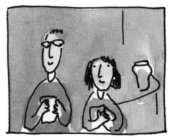

Buy three packets of crisps for the journey.

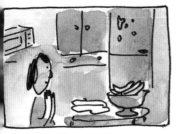

Back in Sussex, I feel emotional to see the same old stuff when everything else is so different.
Same old bowl of bananas.

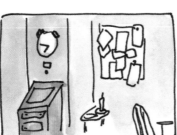

Same old clock with a bit of tinsel on it, same old crowded noticeboard.

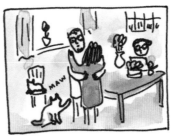

Same silly old cats.
'Ahh, Mikey, so good to see you.'
Mum goes on laptop behind bunches of snapdragons.

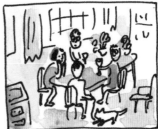

Dinner round our long table.
'Mikey, could you get the yoghurt? I've blocked myself in.'

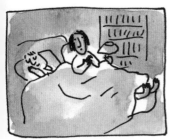

Wake up at 2 in the morning, my hands and feet are burning.

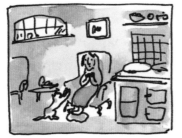

Sit by the Aga in Mikey's Slanket, holding frozen slices of bread with a frozen ham under my feet.
'Go away, stupid cat.'

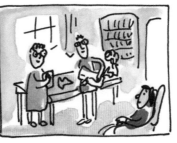

In the morning, Mum and Tom open my presents for me (hands too painful to do it).
'A nice cushion from Granny.'
'And a bag of plastic sea creatures, lovely!'

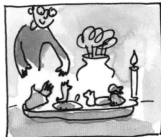

Mum makes an Easter garden out of the sea creatures and her fossil collection.

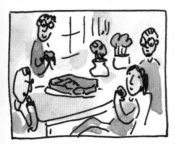

She's also made a discreet cinnamon birthday cake. Decorating it seemed inappropriate. We all have some and avoid singing 'Happy Birthday'.

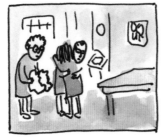

I haven't seen Granny and Grandpa since Christmas, they bring me some comfy slippers with pompoms on.
'Ahh, darling.'
'Thankyou, wonderful slippers!'

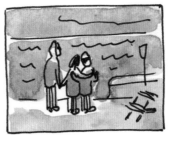

By Sunday, my feet feel a bit better. Me, Tom and aunt Lucy go to the beach at Felpham. It's FREEZING.
'Everything smells better here, creosote, seaweed, salt...'

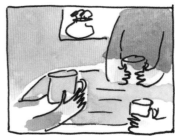

We walk down the promenade for about a minute then go to the Boathouse Cafe.
'Mm, Bovril and melamine.'

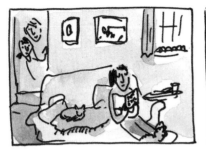 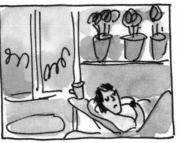 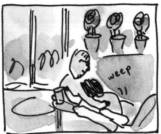 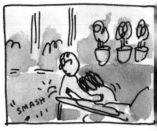

Lots of relatives are around as it's Easter weekend. I don't feel very sociable.
'Hey Mat, how ya doin'?'
'Fine thanks, reading a book about genocide in Darfur.'

Go and lie around in the conservatory. Love the smell of geraniums in there. I feel upset more often now that weird symptoms have started to appear.

Mikey comforts me.
'It's funny, you try so hard to protect your children from harm, then there are things you just can't protect them from.'

My glass falls on the floor.
'Ah dear, I'll clear that up later.'

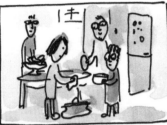 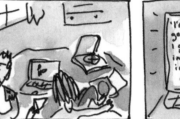 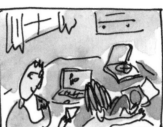 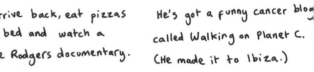

The next day, pack our stuff up to go back to London.
'Some homemade soup...'
'Why don't you take this papaya as well?'

'Bye, Mumma, love you.'
'Bye, Tom, thanks for everything.'
I don't want to go.

Arrive back, eat pizzas in bed and watch a Nile Rodgers documentary.

He's got a funny cancer blog called Walking on Planet C. (He made it to Ibiza.)

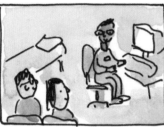 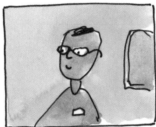 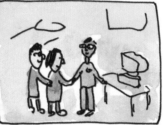 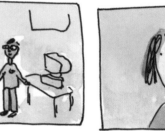

That week, me and Mum go for a meeting with the surgeon. He's very caring and talks to us for a long time. I ask how big the tumour was.

'As big as an apple.'
I wonder what kind of apple. Cox's Pippin? Granny Smith?

'Great to see you looking so well, Matilda. See you again soon.'
His wife is having her first baby in a couple of weeks.

'Oh lovely, congratulations!'

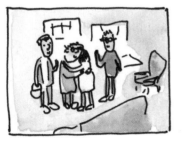 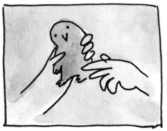 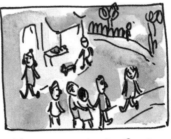 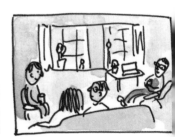

Lucy and my dad, James, come to visit.

James gives me a marble owl.
'Whoops, left the price on.'

We walk to London Fields.
'It's like being on a university campus, all these young people, very nice.'
I notice someone I sort of know and am grateful that we mutually blank each other.

Back at home.
'Beautiful sky out there.'
(It was beautiful.)

APRIL

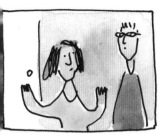

'My shit's gone bright yellow. Just splashed myself in the face with it.'
'Ah dear. Wanna go to the park?'

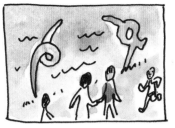

It was a lovely day.
'Even those turdlike sculptures look nice.'

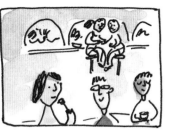

Share a cheesecake in the café. Sweaty, healthy runners smooching by the window.

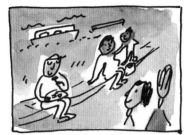

A man sitting on the pavement eating a plate of bacon and eggs in the sun.

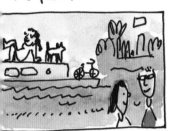

Sexy woman drifts past on a canal boat with a cat and a pink and orange racing bike.
'Ha! All the cool things!'

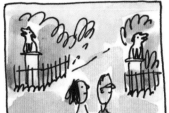

Dogs of Alcibiades guard the entrance to the park.
'They look like they don't know what's going on.'

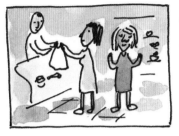

On the way back I buy a big bag of bones to make marrowbone soup, good if you're having chemo, apparently. A woman is telling the butcher about her holiday in Costa Rica.
'Ooh it was lovely... you go first, darlin, don't mind me.'

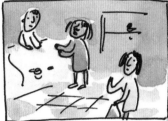

'My husband's got heart failure, I've just had cancer so we thought we'd go for seven weeks. Nice bit of veal, please.'
'I've got cancer, that's why I'm buying these bones!'

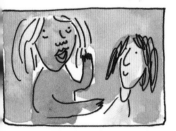

'You get to Costa Rica, there's a yellow spotty fruit there, cancels out all your chemo symptoms. And get down to Peckham if you need a wig, they'll sort you out. This isn't my real hair, wouldn't know it wouldya!?'

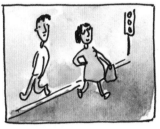

She was very nice. A man eyes me up and I enjoy sticking my pregnant bump out.

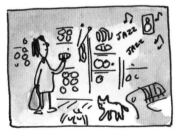

Stop at trendy wool shop. Giant knitting needles and jazz.
'Would this wool be alright for a baby?'

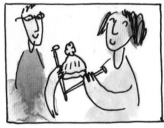

That evening, I knit a tiny hat. It's the only baby thing we've got!
'Bobble's a bit big.'

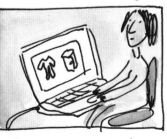

Then panic buy a load of Babygros on the internet.
'Swaddling wrap?'

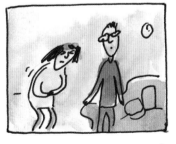

'I have no idea what I'm doing.'

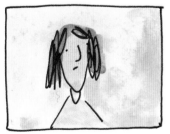

Later, shit's still yellow and stomach cramps get really bad.
'How much are they expecting you to put up with?'

'I dunno, quite a lot I think.'

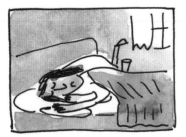

The next day I have an appointment with my oncologist. I feel terrible, still got cramps and feel shivery and weak.

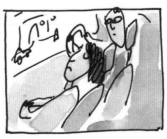

Very glad to still have Mum's car so I don't have to get the bus.

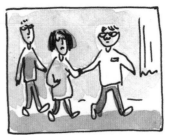

My favourite nurse leads me by the hand to a chair for a blood test. 'You look tired, Matilda.' 'Yes, I don't feel that good.'

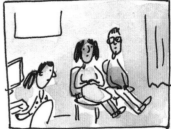

Update the oncologist about my symptoms. 'I got the weird painful hands and I've had stomach cramps and diarrhoea for about 5 days, had to get up 10 times in the night.'

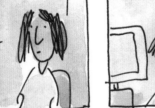

'May I be very rude?' 'Yes, please do.'

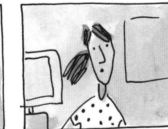

'Why didn't you phone the chemo hotline if you were worried about these things?'

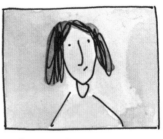

'Um, I dunno really. I thought they might be normal chemo symptoms that'd go on their own.'

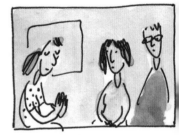

'Please, always, always, always phone the chemo hotline in future.' 'OK. I will.'

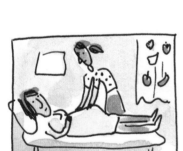

Quick examination. 'Nice and soft.'

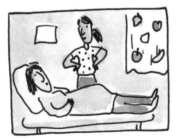

'Now, tell me, do you like spiders?' 'No!'

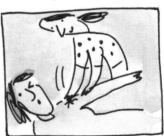

'Good, neither do I.' 'Eeek!' She heroically squashed a big spider crawling up my arm.

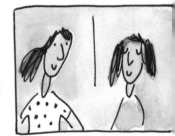

'It wasn't that big.' 'I think it was quite big.'

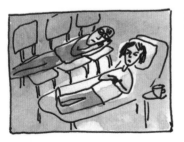

She suggests a night in hospital to monitor my symptoms. Cramps every 10 mins or so. Tom sleeps on 3 chairs lined up in a row.

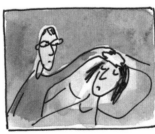

And sponges my forehead when my temperature goes up.

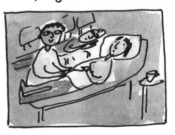

The doctors are worried the cramps might be labour pains. A kind midwife looks after me all night. 'We'll send you back to the baby unit in the morning, okie kokie, my love?'

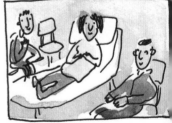

Some sweet ambulance men wait with me while my prescription arrives. We compare scars. 'I'm looking forward to wearing a bikini and showing mine off.' 'Got this one on my neck, tell everyone a shark did it.'

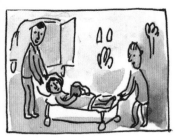

Taken by stretcher to the ambulance.
'You keep hold of your handbag, sorry, it's a bit bumpy, isn't it?'

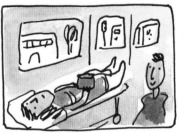

It's odd to see the top of Hackney Road going backwards. Ambulance man asks about my job.
'I'm a teacher, art, 18-year-olds, yes, it's great.'
'Well, as long as it's something you love.'

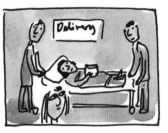

I wonder why I never want to say 'I'm a lecturer in animation and children's writer' which is what I am.
'Matilda Tristram, where's she supposed to be?'
'Ah, one minute please.'

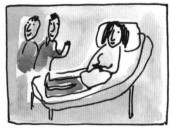

Taken to a side room, sad to see the ambulance men go.
'You stay positive, darlin, ok?'
'I will, thanks, bye-bye.'

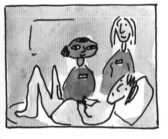

'You're a tiny bit dilated, sweety, so it's possible they're labour contractions.' This hospital has a good reputation for looking after premature babies.

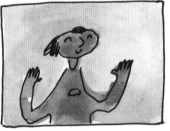

'One was born at 24 weeks recently and he's fine!'
I'm 26 weeks, the nurses seem excited.

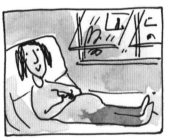

My side room is very nice, I can smell the rain and see wet yucca plants and an upside-down wheelbarrow.

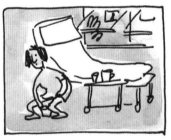

The doctors want me to collect my wee in a jug. I leave the curtains open and don't care who can see me from across the quad.

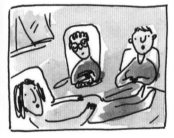

Me and Lucy talk about Thatcher's funeral (the next day), Mum does some knitting and falls asleep.
'10 million pounds!?'
'So disgusting.'

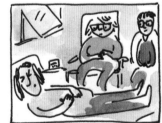

Polly brings some chocolate ginger bites. Delicious but make my stomach cramp.
'I don't think it's labour pains.'
'Poor Mat.'

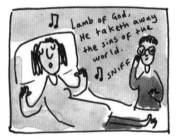

I sing a bit of a Catholic mass by Frances Mary Hunter Gordon that I like and Mum cries.
(Written in a folk style in 1967 when FMHG was 15.)

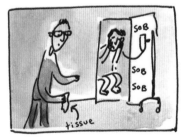

Tom arrives just as I spray diarrhoea all over the bathroom and myself.
'It's everywhere!
I hate this so much!'

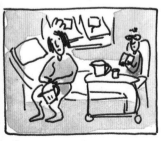

Doctors want me to collect my shit in a jug now, too. Good times.

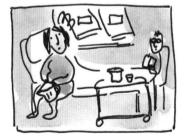

Slightly disappointed there's no one across the quad to see me do it.

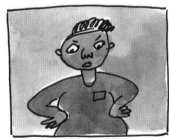

Later, a nurse comes.
'Why are you in your own room??'

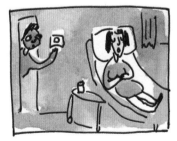

'Because I've got CANCER and I need to not get an infection.'
'Ah, sorry, darling, let me just turn the light off for you.'
She backs out of the door.

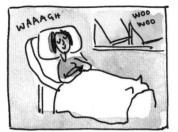
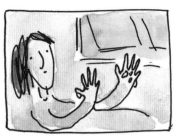
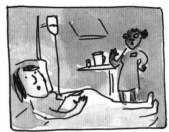
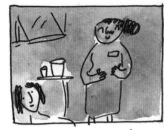

I don't at all mind the sound of screaming babies coming from the ward. I will be glad when mine screams because he'll be alive. They sound like birds. There's a wood pigeon in the tree outside. Lovely sound.

My hands are still sore from the last chemo dose. The skin is peeling off like it's been burnt. I worry that I won't be able to feel my baby's skin properly when he's born.

In the middle of the night, a different nurse comes. We talk about the government and things. 'Of course they're not buying flat-screen TVs, they can't afford to eat or heat their houses!' 'Terrible, the inequality!'

She tells me she had a gastric obstruction once and that labour pains are nowhere near as bad. Sort of comforting.

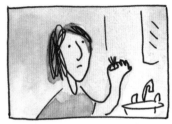
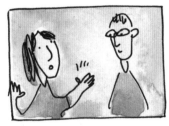
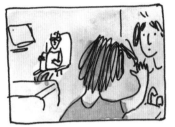
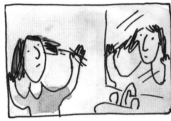

In the morning, I notice my pubes and armpit hair are falling out.

'Damn, I'm not fighting the patriarchy any more.'

Head hairs seem to be staying put for the time being.

A few more strands than usual fall out when I run my fingers through it.

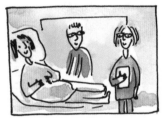
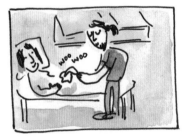
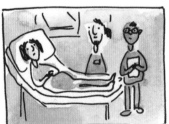
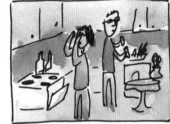

Lovely doctor from the pain team has heard I'm back in hospital and comes to see me. 'Sorry to see you and nice to see you! How are things?' Comforting to see familiar faces.

I'm surprised by how many male midwives there are. Nifty blue pyjamas and orange Crocs. One listens to the baby again. Sounds like one of the wood pigeons is in there too.

They conclude that it isn't labour, most likely chemo side-effects or an infection. 'You can go when your white blood cell count is back to normal.' (Normal is 1, mine is 0.2.)

I'm allowed home when it gets to 0.5. Cry about tiny things. 'Can't be bothered to cook dinner, boo hoo hoo.' 'You sit down and I'll do it.' (Sweet potato and peanut butter gratin.)

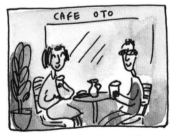
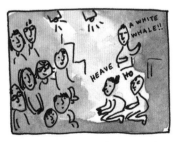
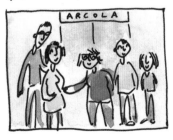
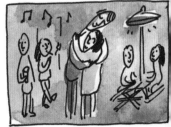

I'm given a week off chemo for things to settle down. It feels like a holiday. 'All my favourite writers lived through something shit; George Orwell, Primo Levi, Kurt Vonnegut...' 'Know what you mean.'

Go to see Moby Dick at the theatre with family. Lots of good pretend rowing.

Everyone admires my bump. 'So exciting, little chap!'

Later, we go to two pubs and a party. I can tell who knows what by how hard I'm hugged. 'Ah, Matilda, great to see you out!' It's good to sit under outdoor heaters with friends.

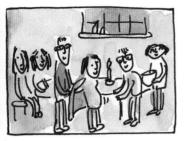

Later that week we go for dinner at Matt and Ruth's. A beautiful flat in a converted abbey with woods around it.
'Ahh! Proper little basketball these days, isn't he!?'

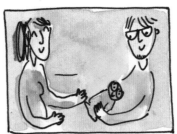

'Sorry, we got you a marble owl then I read your comic and saw you'd already got one!'
'I can't get enough of marble owls!'

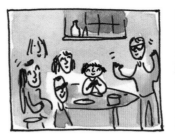

Laugh so hard I feel some internal stitches burst.
'And they carried this sloth across the road, he looked like he thought he was flying, so serene!'

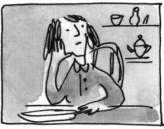

When conversation goes quiet I wonder if everyone's thinking about me having cancer. Perhaps they are. But that's OK.

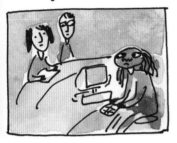

Go for another baby scan. Very unfriendly receptionist.
'I told you to put the folder over there and not queue up.'
I want to shout
'FUCK YOU I'VE GOT CANCER!'
(and I'm still being friendly).

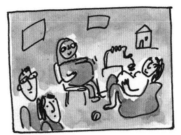

Am annoyed by other pregnant women in the waiting room.
'I feel so tired, my mum was like "pregnancy's not a disease you know" and I'd just had a baked potato so of course my blood sugar was up. Should've had my cervix stitched shut at 14 weeks...'

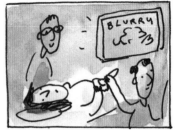

'Should've had your mouth stitched shut, more like.'
'He he.'

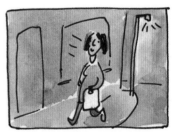

Forgot to wear contacts so can't really see anything this time.
'He's looking sturdy, good.'

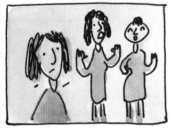

People say that having cancer makes them more peaceful and tolerant.
'Oh, but the Kindle will NEVER replace the book.'

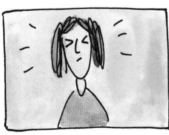

I'm finding the opposite is true. I don't know how long I've got left! Can't waste any time on these boring conversations!

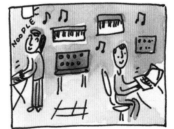

I go and do music with my friend, Tim. Haven't for months. We've almost done enough for an EP. It's fun!
'Yeh that's sounding good.'

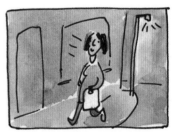

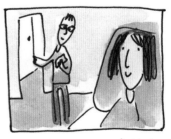

He gives me a copy of a record I did backing vocals on. It feels great walking home in the dark and not wearing a coat.

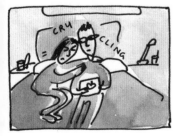

That night I feel upset.
'I don't wanna die, I wanna do so many more projects!'
'Sure you won't die.'

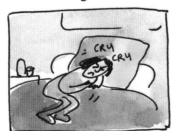

'And I keep getting emails advertising disposable clothes!'

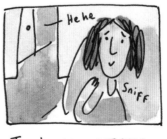

Tom laughing at Twitter in the loo cheers me up.
'Whatcha laughing at?'

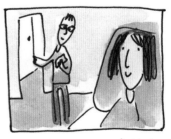

'Noel Gallagher said that Liam is such an angry man he's like a fork in a world of soup.'
'Aw.'

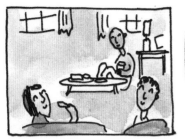

Adam and Alan come over, Alan brings lots of cakes; cheesecake, tiramisu, fruit custard. We talk about baby names.
'Eric is cute.'
'Mum's already calling him Joe.'

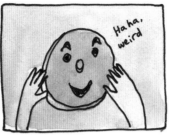

There's also a mad-looking giant jammy dodger.
I eat the eyes and nose.

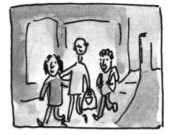

Alan's just moved back to London from Florence for a great new job as an accessories designer.
'They're putting me up in Pimlico, I'll see if I can sneak you into the spa.'

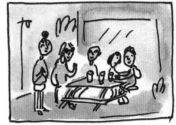

We have orange juices outside. People Alan knows pass by, just like he wanted.
'Alan, ciao!'
'Hey, Sigrid!'
Adam goes off to the gym.
'Bye, Mats, again soon, yeh?'

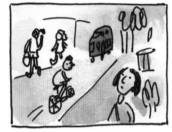

The next day I go for a blood test before my next chemo appt. Another lovely day. All the cool dudes out on their bikes in shorts.

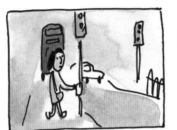

My bus is coming.

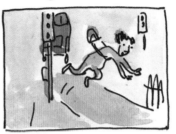

I make a run for it and trip spectacularly in the middle of the road.

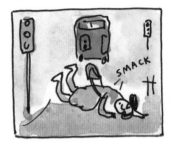

Land on my face, hands and pregnant bump.

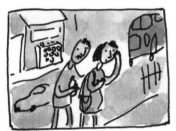

Man runs out of the corner shop and helps me off the road. Cars start driving again.
'You OK, darlin? You have nasty fall!'
'Yes, I'm pregnant, I think I landed on it.'

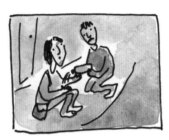

Sit on the pavement outside the dentist, he washes my bleeding hands with a bottle of Volvic.
'You better go hospital I think, darlin, OK? Cut your face as well.'
'Ow, yes, I think so, sorry, so silly of me.'

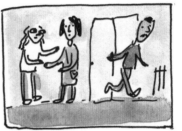

Dentist's receptionist gives me some plasters.
'You be OK to get to the hospital?'
'Yes, I only live over there, I can get a taxi.'

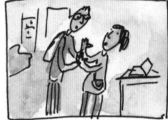

About to order a taxi when Tom gets back from work.
'You're back! Just fell over in the street and landed on the bump, gotta go to hospital!'
'Oh look at your hands, let's go there now.'

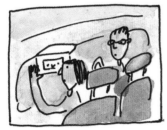

'Gonna have a proper shiner as well.'
Drive to hospital.

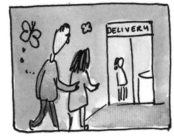

'They're going to be sick of the sight of me in here.'

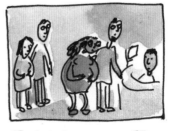

The lady before me is 38 weeks pregnant and has just fallen over too. She looks to be in much more of a bad way than me.
'Do you have her blue folder?'

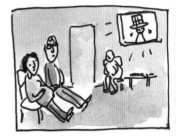

A money-saving programme is on in the waiting room.
'How to make an awful hat for 2 pounds! How to cut a top in half!!'

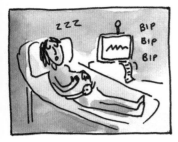

Hooked up to a baby monitor thing for an hour and fall asleep.

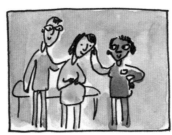

Everything seems OK and we can go.
'Think you broke your fall with your face! No more running for you, my dear, slowly, slowly, OK?'

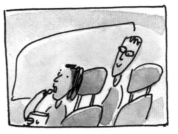

Scoff plantain crisps in the car on the way home.
'Let's have some.'

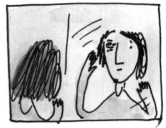

Admire my black eye and cut chin while Tom makes a pasta bake.

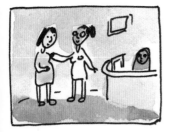

Make it to the cancer unit the next day without injury.
'Dear oh dear, what have you been doing, Matilda?!'
'I was running to catch a bus here.'
'Tut tut.'

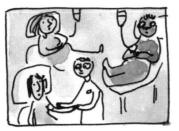

Blood test in the chemo room. One woman is reassuring another about PICC lines.
'Now it just feels like part of me.'
(Mine still feels annoying.)

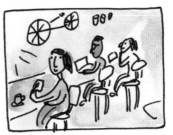

Stop at hip bike/coffee shop on the way home and sit in the sun with a chelsea bun and a chai, pretending to be a normal freelancer.

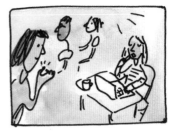

Hot raisins and girls in stripy tops putting on lip balm.

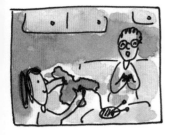

In the morning, Mum arrives to take me to chemo.
'Been knitting a cardigan, bit lumpy and one sleeve's bigger than the other.'
'Haha, lovely!'

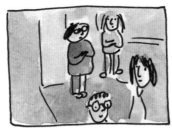

I work out why people stand right by the door of the lift in the mornings...

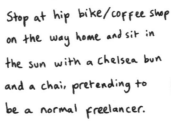

It's so they can run to the nice comfy chairs by the window in the chemo room!

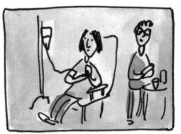

I got the dud normal chair that time. Read about privatisation of the NHS and feel worried. No one would insure me now! Mum brings sandwiches, popcorn, yoghurt, Maltesers and a fruit pot.

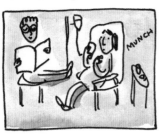

Quick search on some forums shows that the treatment I'm having would cost about $150,000 in the US. Scary.

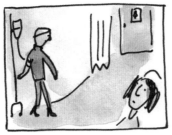

There's another young woman there this time. I think her bald head and turban look quite good. Also with leather jacket and spray-on jeans.

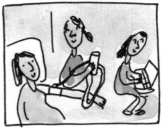

The nurses joke with me about the chemo pump bag.
'Sorry, don't have Prada one for you today, Louis Vuitton next time!'

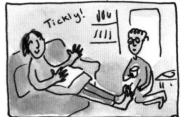

That evening, Mum paints my hands and feet brown with henna. I read online that it helps the painful hand/foot problem.

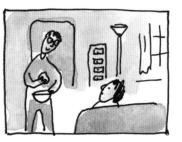

Side-effects aren't nearly so bad this time. The next day is warm and we have mixed mezze outside. I recognise a girl from 6th-form college and hope she doesn't recognise me so I don't have to talk about anything.

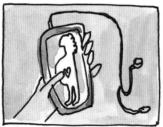

Back at home, Mum makes rye pizza dough.
'Look, it's perfect!'
I'm worried because I haven't felt the baby kick all day.

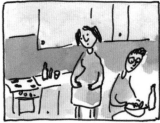

Mum goes back in the kitchen and I download a baby heart monitor app.

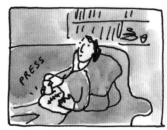

Can't hear anything apart from my own slowly beating heart.

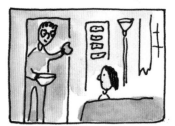

'Do you want to knead it?'
'Not right now.'

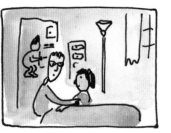

Pizzas go in the oven and Tom gets back from work.
'I'm a bit worried about the baby, he hasn't done anything much all day.'

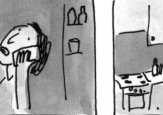

Phone the midwife. She tells me to try drinking something cold.

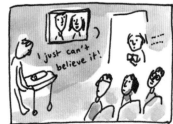

Still nothing.
'Perhaps we should go back to hospital.'

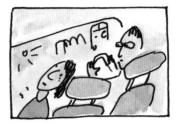

Take the pizzas out of the oven again and drive to hospital.
'Sorry, I will have spoilt the bases.'
It's another beautiful evening. Think if the baby dies I will want to die.

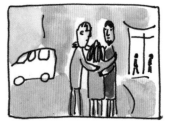

Bump into Jim coming out of A+E while Mum parks.
'Jim! What are you doing here?'
'My ear's about to explode! How about you guys?'
'Just baby stuff, better go...'

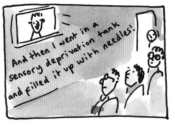

Programme about pointless magic tricks is on in the waiting room.

And then I went in a sensory deprivation tank and filled it up with needles!

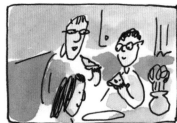

A newborn baby is wheeled past on a tiny trolley, looking surprised. A woman stands next to us, praying.

I just can't believe it!

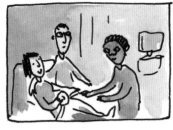

Attached to the monitoring thing again.
'There's his heart beat, he's probably just been facing backwards all day, makes kicking harder to feel!'

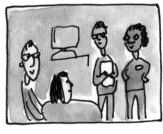

The doctors and nurses are wonderful.
'The truth is, we don't know how chemotherapy affects movement, so please come any time you're worried.'

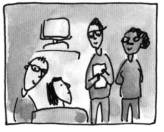

'And how are you coping, generally?'
'Oh, reasonably.'
Always makes me want to cry when doctors ask me that.

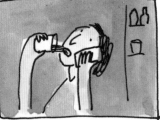

The pizzas are still OK when we get back.
'What a rollercoaster it all is.'
'Slightly undercooked but very nice, eh?'

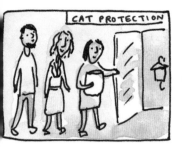

Enjoy a normal afternoon taking a motherload of baby clothes I bought on eBay then decided I didn't want after all, to a charity shop with Claire and Paul.

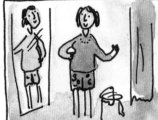

Buy a pair of flowery shorts and a cashmere jumper for £15, bargain.

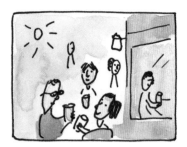

Meet Tom and Matt outside the Jolly Butcher's pub. 'Cor, I miss beer sometimes.' Have an artisan apple juice.

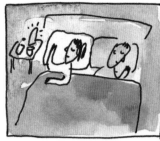

Sleep right through the night for the first time in months.

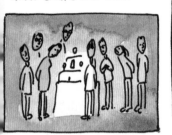

Go to the Ice Age exhibition at the British Museum with Tom and his parents. 'Just exquisite.'

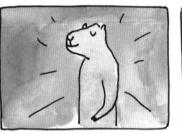

I love the 40,000-year-old half lion half man. 40,000 years!

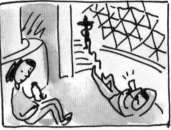

Sit on the floor outside drinking a Yop while a man takes photos of his girlfriend coming down the stairs in a big hat again and again.

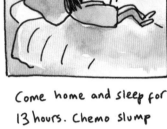

Come home and sleep for 13 hours. Chemo slump or rediscovery of winceyette duvet cover?

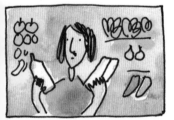

Get a nose-bleed in the veg shop comparing carcinogenic ingredients in non-dairy milk alternatives.

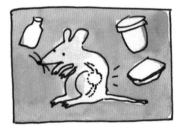

Some of them contain this stuff called carageenan which gives MICE COLON CANCER! It's in everything, ice cream, cream cheese etc.

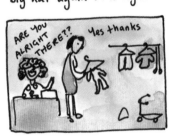

ARE YOU ALRIGHT THERE??   Yes thanks

Go to the boutique baby shop. Predatory shop assistant. Wish I'd bled all over mini Liberty print shorts instead of on the vegetables.

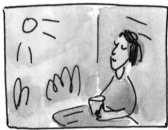

Nose dries out nicely in the sun. Fresh mint tea outside a Turkish caf.

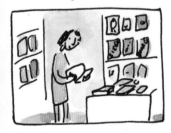

Find a book about tiny handmade homes. Me and Tom had joked that if I die he'd go and live off the grid with the baby in a yurt. I also often fantasise about shipping container homes in fields.

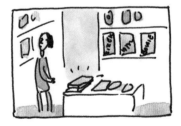

I superstitiously think for a moment that buying the book might mean I'm more likely to die.

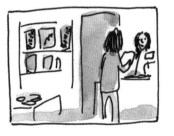

Then decide that's rubbish and buy it after all.

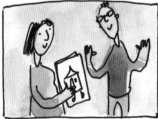

'Got us a present.'
'Coool, tiny homes!'
'We could build one for 2000 quid behind a bush somewhere!'

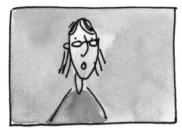

I get touchy when people ask me too many questions. 'So when will they reverse the colostomy?'

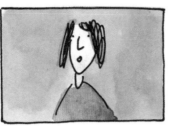

'I don't know, I guess when everything else has settled down a bit.'
Would you normally ask someone about their arsehole so directly?

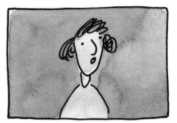

'Does it make it hard to deal with not knowing if the drugs will work?'

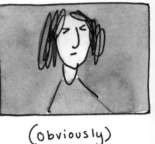

(obviously)

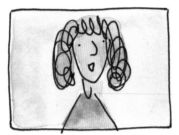

'How's chemo going?'

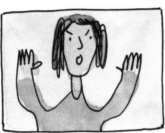

'Oh, just great!'

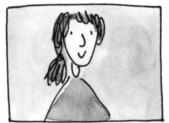

'Did you have a blood test? How was it?'

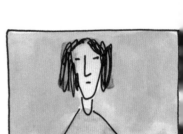

'Fine. Boring.'
Sometimes I don't mind people asking those questions. The ratio of cancer chat to normal chat just has to be right. I don't like to feel like I'm being quizzed.

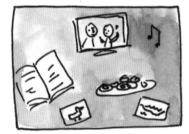

Please, let's talk about something, ANYTHING else, books, films, cooking, holidays, even house prices!

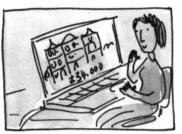

I actually love looking at house prices.
'Ooh, Margate is still cheap, only 30G for a 2 bed flat! Could we live there?'

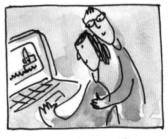

'We'd be "Down From Londons", ruining it all for everyone else.'

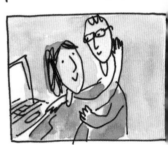

'Think I'd be happy wherever we live!'

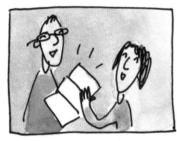

Contract for a children's book me and Tom have been working on for the last year arrives in the post.
'Yess!'
'Our first book!'

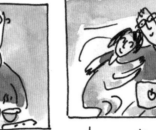

Go out for an Indian to celebrate.
'1.5p per copy each, we've definitely hit the bigtime.'
'Mm, so fragrant, this!'

Life feels good.
'Just got to do a few more books and we'll be sorted!'
Watch Have I Got News For You and fall asleep.

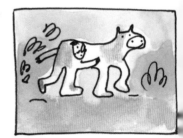

Bad dreams getting sillier. I'm hiding in the arse of a pantomime cow, dropping smoke bombs to avoid going for treatment.

MAY

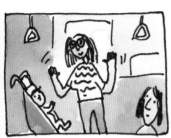

A woman terrorising her baby on the bus home from getting dressing changed.
'WHO'S a bootiful BABY, eh? WHO'S a BOOTiful baby?'

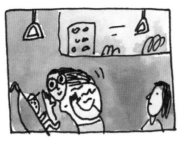

'Hhh? BRRRRR!
Ah? BRRRRR!'
(Jesus Christ.)

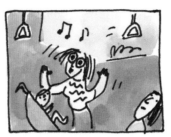

'OLD MACDONALD HAD A FARM, EE I EE I OHH!'

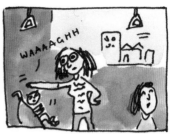

Secretly glad when it cries.

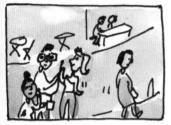

Pass a load of Hackney types on the way to meet Cesca.
'Do you girls wanna hear what's been my day's biggest choon? Take an ear each and have a little boogie, man.'

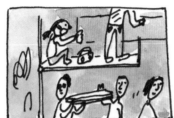

Lots of hot young people sanding the outside of a dark grey pub and carrying planks.

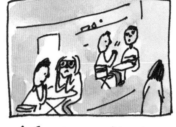

A French girl whingeing;
'I was always ze one never celebrating, never invited...'
Boys talking about making an augmented reality app for Vaseline;
'Gonna blow everything else out of the water.'

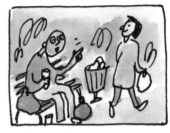

A pissed tramp tells me to 'have a nice day'.
'I will, thanks, you too.'

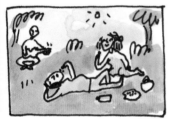

Small things like eating grapes in the park seem significant these days.
Cesca tells me about her woodblock printing class.

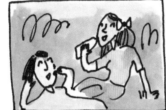

'This retired banker is doing one of his pet rabbit.'
'Ha! So bankers do have hearts after all.'

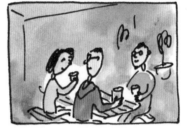

Go to meet Tom and George. More artisan apple juice.
'So are there going to be any steamy scenes in the comic?'
'Nope, no steam whatsoever.'

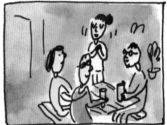

A nice drunk girl comes and congratulates us. I can't remember where I know her from. 'Honestly, I'm so, so happy about the baby.'
'Ah thanks!'
(Ex work-mate of Tom's. I think how much steamier than me she'd probably be at the moment.)

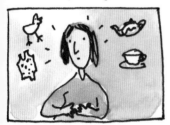

Friends keep offering to arrange baby showers for me.
Not sure how I feel about it. Still can't believe it will be OK and don't really feel like celebrating.

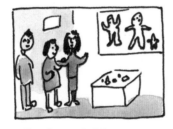

Me, Pia and Edwin go to the Japanese Outsider Art exhibition at the Wellcome Collection.
'We should get together and make freaky dolls for your baby shower!'
A great idea.

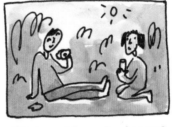

Edwin and I garden hop our way back from Bloomsbury.
'Well, you seem exactly the same, very hardy.'
'Just got to get through the next 5 years without it coming back then I can relax a bit.'

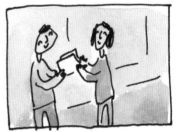

He gives me some drawings as a get-well present.
'Don't open it while I'm here, I'll realise that they're crap!'
'Haha OK!'
(They're excellent.)

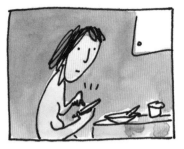

One morning I get stuck reading old Twitter accounts of young, dead bowel cancer patients.

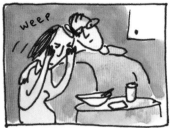

'I'm so frightened.'
'Gotta stop reading those things.'

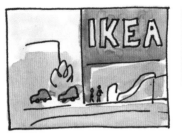

Go to Ikea with Claire to take my mind off it all.

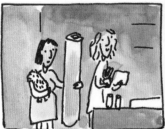

Buy two rugs and some glasses with pineapples on. Claire gets a cushion and a plant.

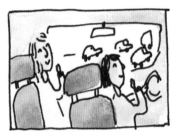

There's a huge traffic jam.
'I love being alive and in a traffic jam!'
We eat lots of spongy Swedish sweets and drink KOLSYRAD APPELDRYCK.

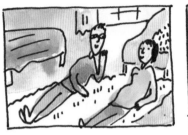

Put the rugs out in our room, cosy.
'I can imagine putting a baby here.'

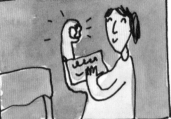

More nice get-well presents arrive in the post.
A folksy pencil case and a rubber peanut. Very me.

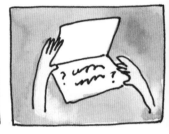

People often write that they don't know what to say. I don't really know what to say either apart from 'Yes, it's shit, isn't it?'

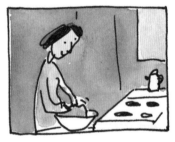

Make some sourdough rye bread.

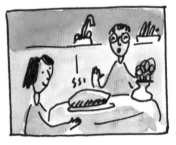

Mum says it looks like a trilobite about to burrow through prehistory.

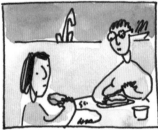

Tell her I've been crying a lot and feeling scared. She says she can't cry.
'I've got a brick wall of tears that won't come out.'
'You can cry through me.'

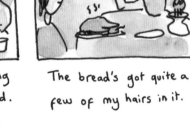

The bread's got quite a few of my hairs in it.

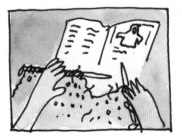

So has my knitting.
(A baby poncho.)

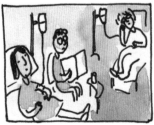

Next chemo dose is quiet and uneventful. Woman opposite is 'bored shitless'.

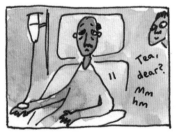

Man in a chair next to me on his own, looking sad. He's got a beautiful long nose, hiccups, and only says 'Mm hm'.

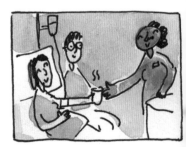

'No sugar for you my darling, sweet enough already.'
(I like that joke.)

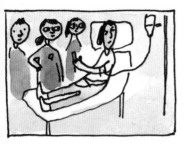

I've got to give myself bone marrow boosting injections after each dose. 'I can't do it!' 'Come on, look at it, it's not so bad, Matilda.' 3 nurses encourage me.

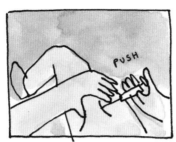

Manage to do it in the end. Hardly hurts at all.

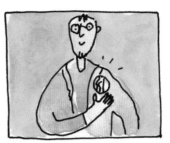

Mikey comes to visit with Beating Bowel Cancer arseless shorts badge from his friend, Denise.

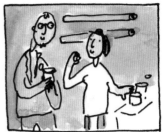

We have a nice time choosing buttons for the baby poncho. 'These are sweet.'

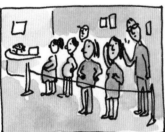

Tom notices a bald bit in my hair when we're waiting to see the obstetrician. 'There, covered it up.'

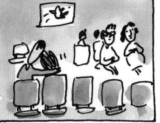

Minor cry about it in the waiting room.

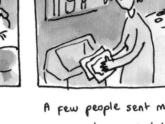

A few people sent me bald head wraps, I threw them straight in the bin.

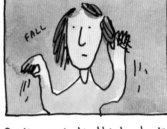

Don't want to think about it until/unless it happens. Will avoid shaving it off for a bit longer.

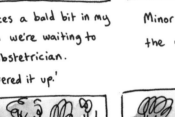

Tom's got time off work and we go to my parents' for the week. I love lying in their garden.

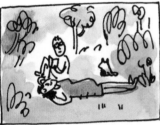

Love it so much it makes me cry (again) in case I die and can't do it anymore. 'So silly, all the nice things make me cry.' 'Better stop doing nice things.' (Ha ha.)

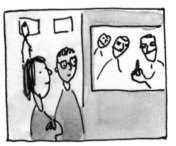

Me, Mum and Tom go to an exhibition of Barbara Hepworth's prints of surgeons in operating theatres in 1948. 'They look like angels, all looking downwards.'

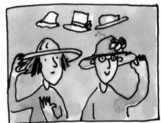

Mum and me try on awful hats (Alex's wedding is soon) while Tom buys pants. 'Bit unnecessarily big.' 'Quite like the flower.'

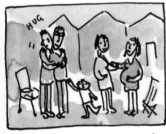

Meet our friends Chris and Julia at Gran and Grandpa's beach hut in Bognor. 'Great to see you guys!' Me and Julia are the same amount pregnant, I'm worried because her bump is much bigger than mine.

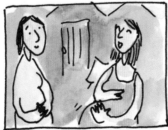

Turns out she's diabetic and has 'massive baby syndrome'. 'Is that an actual thing?' 'Yes!'

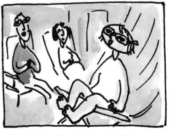

Their 2-year-old, Sam, is very cute. 'Tom, you're gorgeous!' 'Ah thanks, Sam.'

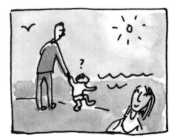

'Can we go and have a lovely time NOW? Throw stones in the sea NOW?' 'Hehe, he's so bossy these days.'

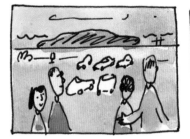
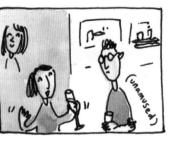
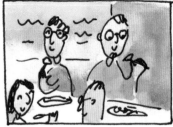
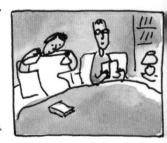

Me, Tom, Mum and Mikey go to a restaurant on Littlehampton beach, affectionately known by locals as 'The Turd'.
'How apt!'

Once I met the young architect who designed it, at a private view of his work (design week).
'Oh! You designed THE TURD! We all love THE TURD!'

Fish and chips, crab linguine and pannacottas for pudding.

Later that evening.
'My pregnant boobs look great at the mo, shame the rest of my body is completely fucked.'
'Ah dear.'

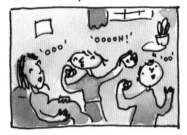
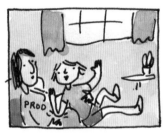
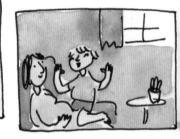
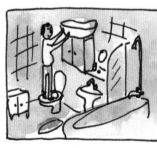

That weekend we go to Tom's parents' for his twin nephews' 5th birthday. They are excitable. Eating Hula Hoops.
'What sound does a Hula Hoop make? OOOOH!'

One has slight baby jealousy.
'Baby in a bump!'
'Don't elbow it or it might fall out!'

Screams his head off when I push him away for trying to wipe snot in my face.
'You pushed me off!'
'There there, keep your bogies to yourself.'

Cheers up again soon after.
'Call the baby Minnie Mouse!'

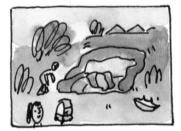
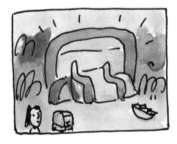
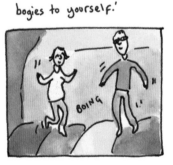
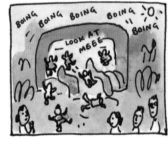

Early next morning I watch the bouncy castle being blown up in the garden in case there's anything funny about it to put in the comic.

There isn't, really.

Me and Tom have a tentative bounce on it before the children arrive.
'I forgot how fun these are!'
'You be careful.'

A very successful party.

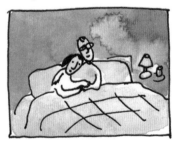
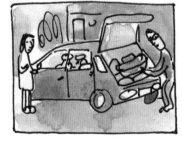
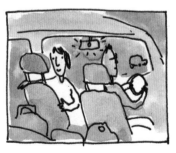
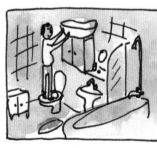

Talk a bit that night about how scary the last few months have been.
'I really thought the baby was a goner...'

I feel emotional to see our car loaded up with donated baby stuff.
'Shit's getting real.'

View of spectacular sunset from the M1 over Northampton.

Deposit baby stuff around the flat.
'Is it OK to change a baby on the floor?'

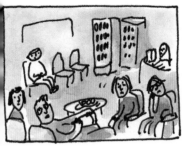

Long wait for pre-chemo blood test with a lot of complaining people. 'I had to wait 2 hours and my arm swelled up like a plum, and my brother died in this hospital.'

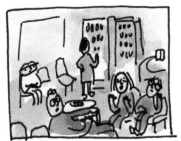

I pretend to go and look at the vending machines... '...all the way from Chingford bla bla bla.'

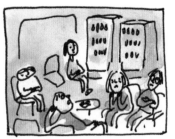

... and sit somewhere else. 'Been here since 2, my appointment was at 2.30...' 'Gordon Bennett, it's always like this.' (It isn't.)

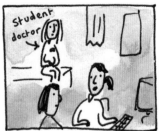

Oncologist thinks the next dose of chemo should be my last before being induced in 3 weeks' time, 5 weeks early. 'Don't want you to accidentally give birth too near to a dose.' (Risk of infection.) 'OK, yup, sounds good.'

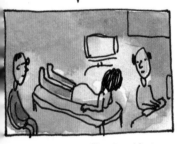

Obstetrician thinks that sounds fine too. 'Looks like he'll be about 4 pounds, very respectable.'

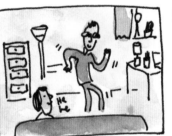

Back at home, Tom does anticipating the baby dance. '3 weeks, OMG!'

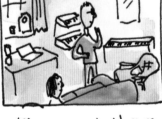

'Maybe we should move some of the synths.' 'Naah.'

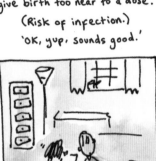

Me and Mikey buy some ultra-tiny Babygros online. 'Run out of boys' stuff.' 'Pink spots and owls'll be alright!'

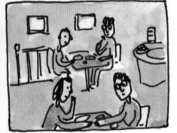

Me and Mum go for lunch at Georgian cafe. I nearly cry thinking about how much I'm going to cry when the baby's born. Mum deftly changes the subject.

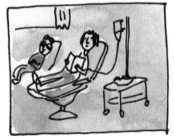

'Must tell you about this amazing dance show I saw with Hannah. The dancers had wigs like the foamy bit of a microphone.'

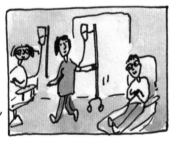

Next chemo session is 6 of 12, half way through! A good milestone. Dose has been raised again after 2 at 20% lower, dreading painful hands and diarrhoea. (Mum asleep in massage chair.)

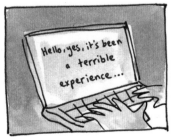

Dragging my drip to the loo, I get lots of soppy looks for being so pregnant. It's quite nice.

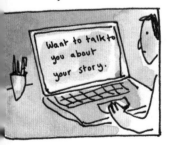

There are a couple of cancer euphemisms that I feel need debunking. First, it's not a 'story' it's real!

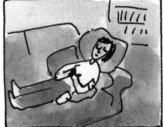

Nor is it my 'journey'. I'm not going anywhere.

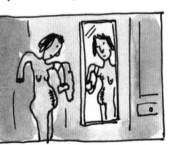

Not to mention 'battling'. It's just my body doing strange things.

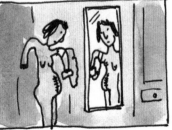

I prefer to describe it like this.

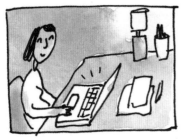

Enjoy being called a 'FUCKIN' BALLER*' by someone on an American comics blog.
* 'Baller': Really cool dude.

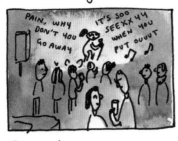

The band are WONDERFULLY TERRIBLE!
'Hee hee, perhaps not very sexy to sing "SEEXXYY" like that.'
'I feel bad slagging off bands, at least they tried.'
'Yes, well done them.'

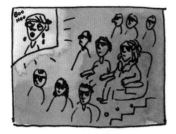

Go and see The Great Gatsby with Mum and Cesca.
Could've shaved about half an hour off if Leonardo Di Caprio didn't have to say 'old sport' quite so many times.

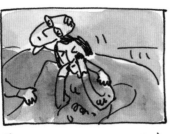

Then remember I've just had 3 months of chemo and now I've got to give birth then have another 3 months of chemo and cry even more.

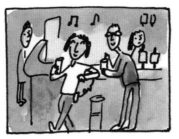

Me and Tom go to a gig at the pub round the corner. I've got white gloves on full of moisturiser and chemo pump dangling round my waist.
'I AM a fuckin' baller!'
(Glass of Appletiser.)

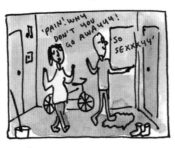

Quite catchy despite being so terrible.

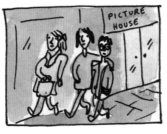

Get bored and leave early.
'Great Crapsby.'
'Heh.'

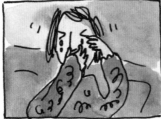

Luckily, my jumper's so cosmic I can wipe my nose all over the sleeves and get away with not washing it afterwards.

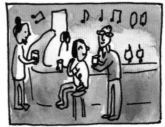

Man with a beard and a bun. Mum had been surprised by the prevalance of this look in East London.
'Hm, yes, I'm not sure about men with buns, it's a bit louche and forthcoming.'
'Yeah, it basically means "hey girls, you can stick your finger up my bum if you like".'
'He he he.'

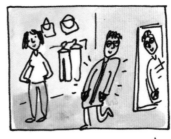

Next day, Mum comes and we go on a consolatory chemo shopping bender.
'Love this jacket!'

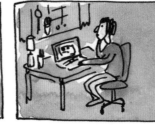

Pass a hospice on the way home and feel freaked out.

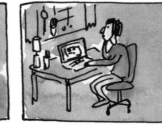

Look at 'elegant al fresco dining accessories' online. Dunno why, no garden and coldest spring for 30 years.

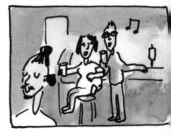

Then we see a man with a beard and TWO buns!
'What does the second bun mean? Aargh!'

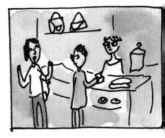

Sweet shop girl asks how the pregnancy has been.
'Quite shit because I've been having chemotherapy the whole time ha ha!'

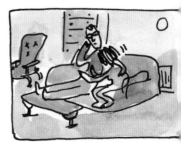

Colossal cry all over Tom's shirt.
'Sure you won't ever have to be in one of those places.'

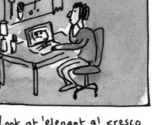

'I do not need a Breton cool-bag or a half-price vintage-style hamper.'

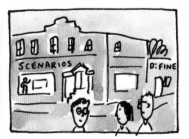

Go to Alex's wedding in Essex. Mum's booked us into a bar/hotel called Scenarios, frosted glass, sexy women on the windows.
'Yup, this is it.'

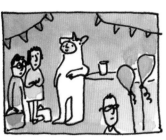

There's a cancer fundraiser on at the bar that night. The staff are all wearing animal onesies and preparing to shave their heads.
'Two rooms, was it?'

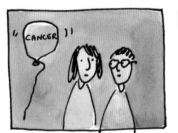

Feel like I'm being followed by Macmillan cancer balloons.
'Cancer in my face everywhere I go scenario.'
'Sorry, darling.'

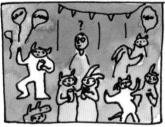

Mikey arrives at midnight and finds his way through the onesies.
'Any idea how to get to the chalets?'

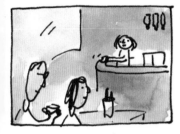

At breakfast, the bar woman tells us about the fundraiser.
'We had a party last night because one of our barmaids has got cancer. Shaved her head because it'll all fall out anyway.'
'Poor thing, funnily enough I'm being treated for cancer too at the moment.'

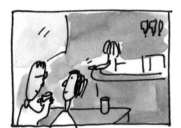

The woman is on cancer-talk autopilot and doesn't hear me.
'Yes, she's very young, but they say it's treatable, still, she's got her friends and family around her.'

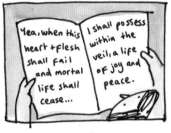

Yea, when this heart + flesh shall fail and mortal life shall cease...

I shall possess within the veil, a life of joy and peace.

At the wedding I have to stop singing during Amazing Grace because the words are making me cry.

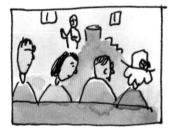

Quiet weep during the prayer...
'Jesus is alive today, if you ask for his help he will help you.'
Because I don't believe a word of it.

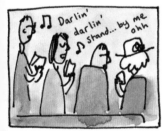

♫ Darlin' darlin' stand... by me ohh

Fine during Stand By Me.

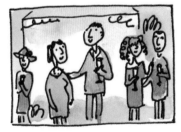

People are surprised to see that I don't look like I'm dying.
'But you look really well?!'
'I know, confusing, isn't it?'
'Your hair hasn't fallen out!'
'It doesn't, always. It is getting a bit thin if that's any consolation.'

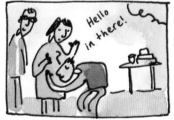

Dangerous bump touching. A man unwittingly rubs his face on the colostomy bag. Bit weird.

Hello in there!

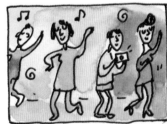

Small dance to ESG.

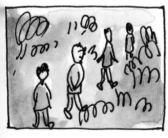

Beautiful countryside walk with Mum, Mikey and Tom on the way home.
'I want to be at the back so I don't have to set the pace.'

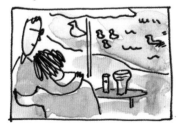

Watch ducklings with a coke and half a shandy.

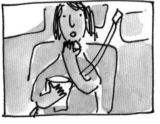

Eat a load of marshmallows in the car in the hope they'll stop me getting diarrhoea. (Read it on a forum, seems to work.)

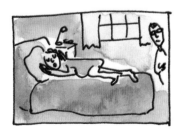

Fall asleep as soon as we get back.
'Want any macaroni cheese?'
'Zzzz.'

JUNE

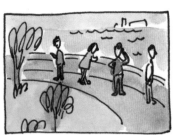

Walk to King Edward's Park in Limehouse with Tom's parents.
'I'd live in Rotherhithe, so much airier by the river.'
'What a lovely park.'

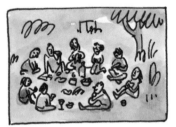

Spend Sunday in Haggerston Park with friends, making more freaky dolls for the baby. A lovely day under the blossom trees.

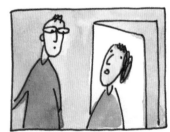

That night, worried I've got another infection.
'Doing weird white shits.'
'Oh dear.'

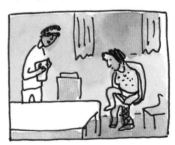

Eventually see a doctor.
'So what do you teach?'
'Art.'
'Aha, I guessed as much.'

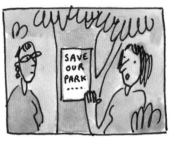

'Oh look, they're going to turn it into a sewage plant. Very Simpsons.'

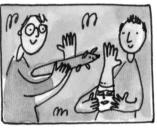

'I think it's a sausage dog' (Matt's).
'Weird hand with a blindfold on' (Edwin's).

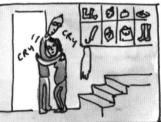

'Maybe we should go to hospital again, could do without an infection so close to giving birth. I want my old body back.'

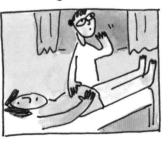

I tell him about everything.
'Gosh, it really makes you think about your own mortality, doesn't it?'
'Er, yes, yes it does.'

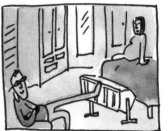

We put the cradle, made for Tom and his sisters when they were babies, at the end of our bed. Tom can rock it with his foot from anywhere in the room.
'Useful long legs!'

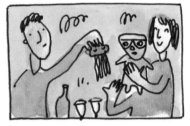

'Run out of steam with this jellyfish' (Adam's).
'An alien with glasses!' (mine).

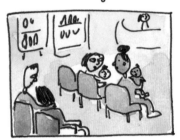

Wait around in A+E. Two girls talk about nothing but their babies for 4 hours.
'Sometimes, when I think he's smiling, he's actually doing a poo! Aren't you, precious?'

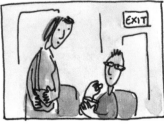

'They said it's not an infection and I should give myself an enema.'
'Oh good.'

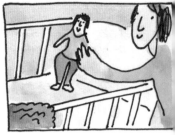

Put in a woolly blanket and a doll of myself that I made (so if I die I'll still be there).

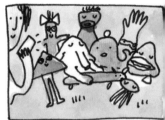

'What a lot of freaky new mates he'll have!'
'Take a picture!'
'Trust Alan to make one with a weird sexy mouth!'

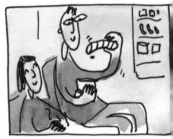

Happy vending machine incident:
'My corn snacks knocked out a flump*!'
'Hehe, I am knocking out flumps.'
*flump: A long, floppy white marshmallow.

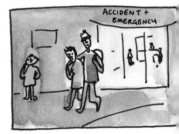

'What a life.'

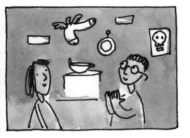

Go to Pompeii exhibition at the British Museum with Mum. 'How interesting, a penis with a penis!' (An oil lamp.)

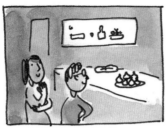

'I like that the penis is a protective symbol rather than an aggressive one.' 'Look at those carbonised figs, amazing!'

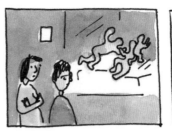

Casts of a family the moment they burnt to death. 'Funny, I imagined them lying still but of course they'd have been moving.' 'So sad...'

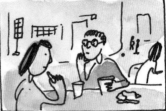

Eat oat biscuits in the cafe and talk about the timing of things.
'It's good, really, that it happened when it did. Any earlier and I'd have had to abort the baby, any later and they mightn't have been able to operate and I could be dead.'
'Yes, "good" in tiny letters, "BAD" in big letters.'

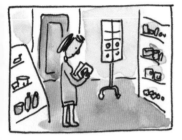

Later that week I spend a long time comparing teats in the chemist. Glad no one asks if I need any help (I do).

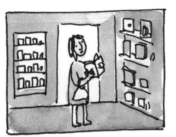

Wander into a bookshop and look at a book about Sun Ra.

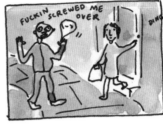

Then wander out again. A man on drugs is shouting. I think about how amazing it is that people can do so many damaging things to their bodies and not die.

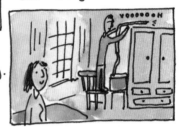

Back at home, Tom is hoovering EVERYTHING. 'So much gunge up here!' 'What shall we do tonight? Our last babyless Thursday?'

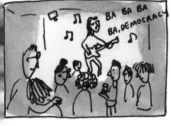

There's another gig on round the corner. Laetitia Sadier from Stereolab. 'I wish I was French.'

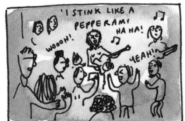

And Viv Albertine from The Slits. Lots of smitten punk blokes. 'So awesome!'

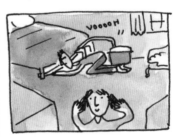

Next day, more hoovering. 'Loads of moths under here.' 'What shall we do tonight? Our last babyless Friday!?'

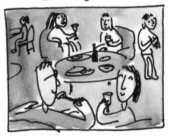

Go out for supper at a busy pub in Farringdon. It's nice to be in that part of town and NOT be going to hospital.

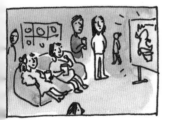

At the weekend, go to an exhibition with Cesca of our friends' films. Boxes of free crisps and old sofas.

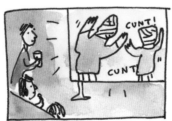

Men with their heads wrapped in clingfilm shouting 'CUNT' at each other.
'I quite like some of their shorter films, think they're online somewhere.'

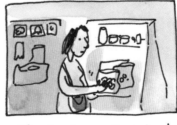

The day before I'm induced I go to Westfield Shopping Centre and wander around John Lewis fingering cotton wool balls and not really knowing what to do.

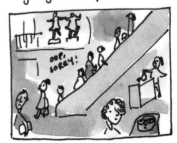

Sleepily lean back against a man's paunch on the escalator.

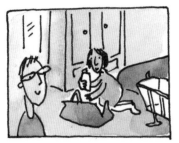

Packing hospital bag. Tom suggests that I don't take BS Johnson's Christy Malry's Own Double Entry to read. 'Nice bit of pessimistic metafiction to welcome the little lad.'

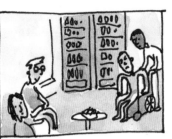

Quick dressing change at cancer unit beforehand. A young-ish very thin man is crying and in pain, not wanting to get in his wheelchair. 'Are you comfortable, Sir?' Sad.

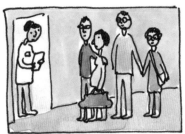

Arrive at the baby ward with Mum, Tom and Mikey. They're not expecting me. 'I've got an appointment to be induced, Matilda Tristram, obstetrician said come here.' 'Sorry, can't see you on the list. Go to the delivery suite, please.'

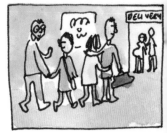

'They ought to have the bunting out, ready!' Keep seeing anxious-looking very pregnant women waddling about. 'Look at that! My bump's so small.'

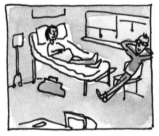

Given a nice HUGE bedroom. 'There's so much space, I feel like I ought to rehearse a monologue or something.'

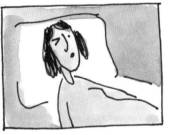

Have the first dose of induction stuff globbed onto my cervix at 9pm. It's not as painful as everyone says it is. 'I am a pain veteran.' The doctor tells us to go and get some dinner.

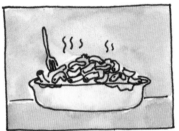

Glob of macaroni cheese with a few bits of veg on top. 'That'll keep me going.'

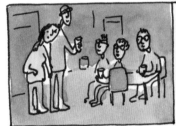

More stuff globbed on my cervix in the morning. Told to go and walk around so the baby's head engages. Find Mum, Tom's mum and Mikey in Costa. 'I think the contractions have started, not sure.' 'You'd know if they were real contractions, darling!'

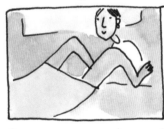

Early afternoon, a different obstetrician comes to see me. 'Well done, you're 1cm dilated, those contractions must've been doing something.'

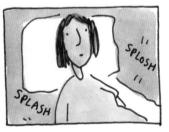

She breaks my waters (not that painful either).

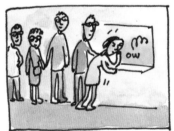

Go and walk around again. Contractions get really painful.

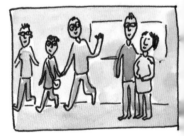

'Um, I feel a bit silly walking around contracting with a big entourage following me about.' 'We'll go and wait in Costa.'

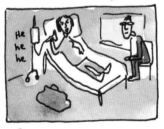

Back in my room, given gas and air for the pain. It makes me laugh. 'Want a go?' 'Yeah go on then.'

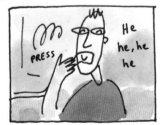

'You just have to press the thing and breathe in.'

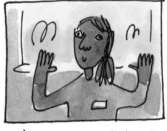

Later, a nurse tells me I'm using it wrongly. 'Don't press it! Just breathe in! You'll gas yourself if you press it!'

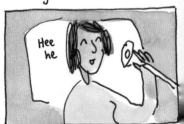

'Whoops, been ODing for about the last hour.'

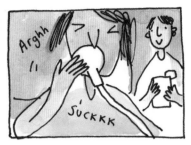

Thought I could do without an epidural but after 7 hours of contractions I've changed my mind. 'Yes, it's only going to get worse, I'm afraid.'

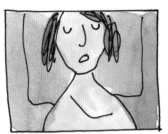

Feel shaky and anxious about being injected in the back. 'You need to keep completely still or I can't do it.' She manages after a few goes.

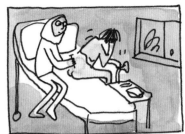

It starts to work and I fall asleep.

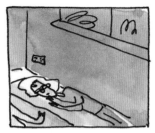

Tom goes to sleep on the floor next to my bed.

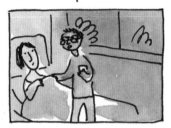

The nurse wakes me up just before 2am. 'Wake up, darling, the baby's heart has dropped, I've just called the doctor.'

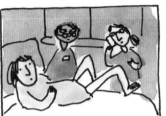

'Only dilated 2cm. Think we need a caesarean.' She phones the obstetrician, who's asleep somewhere in the hospital. 'How quickly can she get here? Is she far away?' 'Not far, dear.'

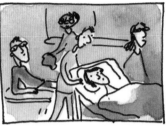

The room fills with people and I'm wheeled off. The nurse wakes Tom up and hands him some blue pyjamas and a hair net. 'We're going in.' 'Going in where? What's going on??'

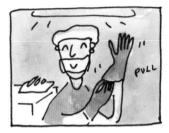

The obstetrician greets us cheerily. 'Ah, hello again, you woke me up!'

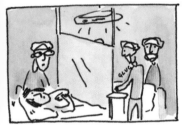

It all happens very quickly and feels like someone rummaging in a handbag. Tom sits next to me. He can see what's happening in the reflection on the lamp.

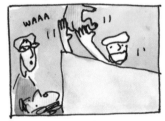

'Here he is!' They lift the baby over my head. I hear him cry and get a good view of his bum. All I can think of to say is 'Wow'.

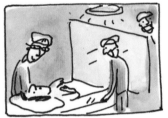

He's having slight trouble breathing and is taken to the Special Care Baby Unit. 'Well done.' 'Is he alright?' 'He'll be fine.'

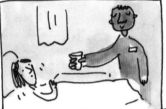

I'm taken to the recovery unit. Being numb up to my armpits makes me claustrophobic. 'I can't breathe, can I have some water?' 'Only tiny sips. Try some deep breaths.'

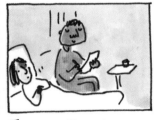

Talk with the calm nurse about Nelson Mandela, who seems like he might die any minute... 'How one man could change the lives of so many...' 'Amazing.'

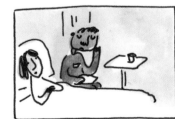

And about my slow diagnosis... 'Terrible, your life they were putting in danger.' (I'm surprised he agrees with me so openly.)

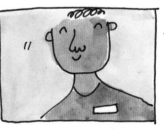

And about our choice of name. 'James like James Bond! He will be strong just like his mother.'

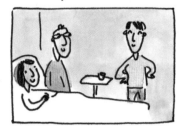

The obstetrician comes and tells me her children love the TV programme I co-wrote. 'They'd be so excited if they knew you were here!' 'Haha, that's excellent!' (I feel much better.)

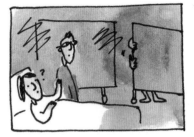

Then taken to a small dark room on the neonatal ward. People in the bay next door wheel some barriers between us straight away. Even darker. 'What did I do?'

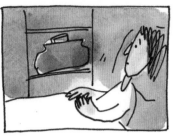

Tom goes to see the baby. I need to sleep but can't until I've seen him too.

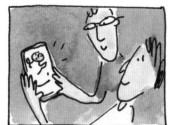

He brings back a photo of him in the incubator. 'He's doing fine, look!' 'Ohh, he's looking right at you! I want to see him so much!'

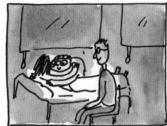

Mum arrives. 'Ahh, Mum, I can't really sit up.' 'Well done, darling.'

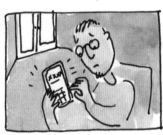

Mikey's not allowed in to see me. (Risk of infection.)

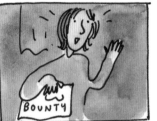

But the Bounty woman is, with a bag of adverts. 'Morning! Can I just give you this Bounty pack?'

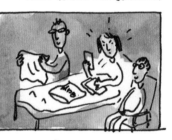

'ISAs, baby photo shoots... surely the Bounty woman is more likely to spread infection by visiting EVERYONE than Mikey is?' 'Another free towel, excellent.'

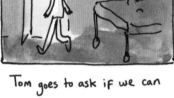

Tom goes to ask if we can have a wheelchair to take me to the baby.

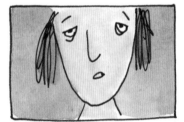

So exhausted but need to stay awake to see him.

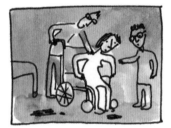

Wheelchair takes hours to arrive. 'Careful, darling.' 'Whoops, bled everywhere.'

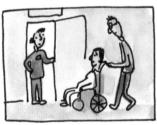

Can't go into the baby unit because the doctors are doing their rounds. 'Come back in an hour.'

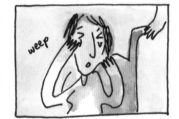

'But he was born 12 hours ago and I still haven't seen him.' 'Sorry, dear.'

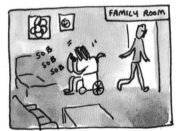

'Do they know I've just had 3 months of chemo and thought he might die?' 'I'll ask them again.' Wondered when I would start crying, surprised I hadn't so far.

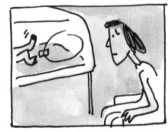

Allowed in at last. It doesn't feel like he's really ours, he could be any old baby in a box. 'Can I hold him?' 'Of course dear, you're the mummy.'

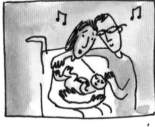

'I can't believe he's OK...' 'Look at his long legs...' We sing him the theme tune from Father Ted, which I often got stuck in my head and hummed a lot when I was pregnant.

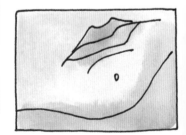

He's got a beautiful dimple in his chin just like Tom. I start to believe it all, slightly.

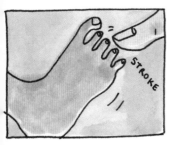

'Look at his amazing toes, I've got a long big toe like that.'

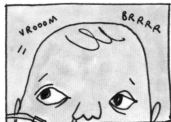

He seems alert and reacts to sounds in the room. 'Look, he recognises my voice!' We make traffic noises so he's used to the cars on Hackney Road when he comes home.

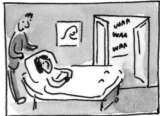

The nurses think I'm crying because I'm worried about the baby. 'Don't worry, Mummy, he'll be OK.' (I'm not worried about him, I'm worried about me!)

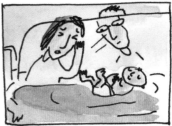

'He's so beautiful... I want to see him grow up.' 'Sure you will see him grow up.'

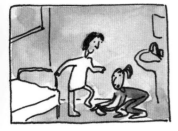

Go back to the ward and sleep until evening.

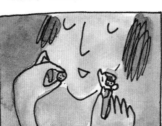

Scoff two packets of fruit pastilles...

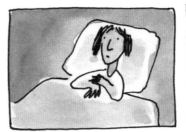

... and a roast chicken dinner (delicious)...

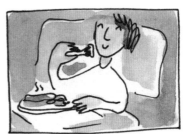

Then moved to the maternity ward.

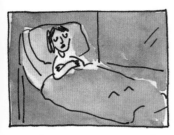

Night nurse tells me all about her mum's cancer and says 60% of getting better is down to your attitude... 'and you're a positive person' (I'm not always, I'm scared shitless most of the time) 'let's get you some new socks' (covered in blood).

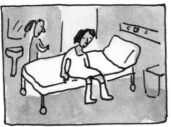

'I'll turn the light out for you, darlin.' 'Thanks.' I have problems with the 'think positive and you'll be fine' platitude.

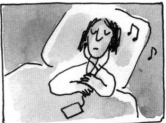

It's as though, if you're not positive all the time you're more likely to die, which makes you feel guilty and more worried about worrying.

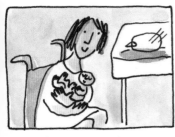

Go and see the baby again the next day and feel a little bit more relaxed.

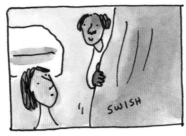

'Have you put him on the breast?' (Breastfeeding nurse.) 'I tried to but nothing came out.' 'We'll see about that.'

As if it's your own fault if you do die. What a load of crap.

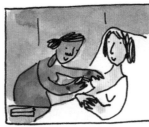

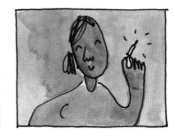

Am expertly milked by another nurse who collects my colostrum (first milk) in pipettes. 'Sorry dear, this might hurt.' 'That's fine, you go ahead.' We compare stories about delayed diagnoses.

She tells me about her son whose skull went rotten once. 'But now he's fine and a footballer!'

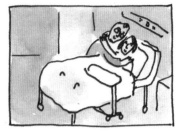

Later, Mikey is finally allowed in.
'Ahh, darling, so good to see you're really OK! Just saw James, he's amazing!'

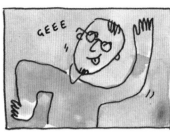

'He went like this...'

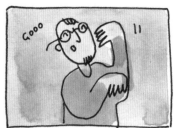

'...and like this...'

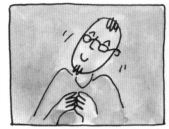

'...and then he stuck his leg out.'

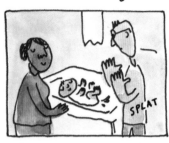

Tom is taught useful tips in the baby unit.
If you stand at the side when you change them, they won't shit up your T-shirt.

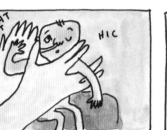

The professional burping technique.

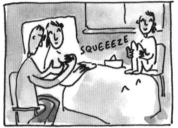

He's better at squeezing colostrum out of my tit than I am.
Hannah comes to visit.
'Hehe, this is funny. Milk whisperer.'

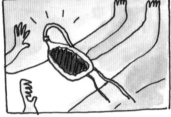

And at getting James to finish his bottle.
'Come on now, lad.'

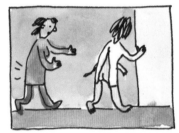

I've had so much weird stuff done to my body I don't care who sees what. Have turned into one of those patients who shuffles along with their bum showing, pursued by nurses trying to cover them up.
'And put some slippers on!'

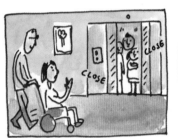

Enjoy being the opposite of a humble invalid.
'Hold the doors! Oh. Screw you guys!'

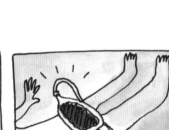

Have a blood transfusion because of low red blood count. Am annoyed because it takes all day and keeps me away from the baby.
'Just a potato for lunch, and they wonder why I'm anaemic!'

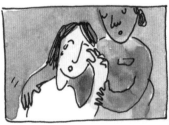

The nurse flops a bag of blood onto my lap while she's changing them over. It reminds me of a heart and freaks me out a bit.

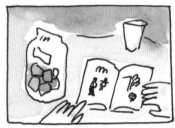

Mum and Mikey give me a packet of fudge and one of my grandmother's tiny sketchbooks.

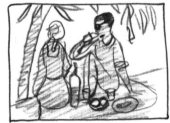

Some brilliant drawings of a holiday to Italy in the 40s.
'Lunch between Rapallo and La Spezia.'
I miss her.

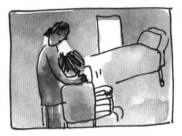

Cry all over the night nurse.
'Don't cry, my dear. It will give the devil a foothold. I have faith; you will get better.'

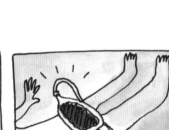

'Thanks.'
I don't mind the God stuff so much any more. It's just another way of saying 'sure it'll all be ok.'

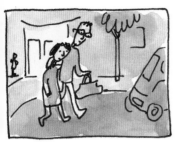

Am checked out the following evening. It feels strange to be leaving without the baby. 'The seasons have changed while I've been in hospital, the air smells flowery and warm at last.'

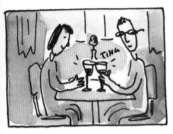

We feed James at 10am and 2pm and treat ourselves to nice lunches in between. 'Cheers to us and James!' 'Best baby ever!'

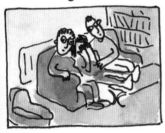

At home that evening, everything seems like too much to cope with. I thought I'd worry less once he was born, but actually I feel more afraid now there's more to lose.

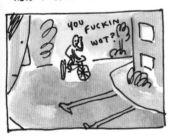

I watch a man cycle slowly round the carpark, swearing his head off down the phone.

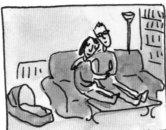

'It's good to be back.'

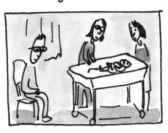

He isn't very good at finishing his bottle. A nurse says he's a 'dozy baby'. 'When do you think he can come home?' 'Mm, not until he's feeding properly.'

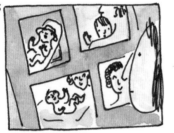

Mum emails some photos of her and me as a baby. I think about how she must be feeling now. Mikey told me she had a nightmare about going down a long dark flight of stairs, at the bottom there was just black nothingness.

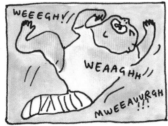

Turns out he's the father of an enormous baby in the tray next to James. He has his leg in plaster and screams non stop the *entire* time. It sounds horrible!

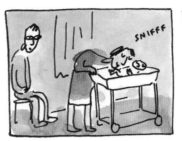

We visit James every day and wait while he sleeps until it's time to feed him. 'Mmm, he smells like oats.'

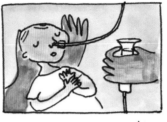

Still has a tube from his nose to his stomach to give him what he can't drink 'He complains a lot less than I did when I had one of those tubes!'

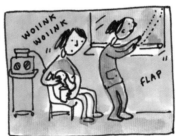

I spend a lot of time in the expressing room, wringing my tits into a machine. 'I'll just close the curtain for you, my dear.'

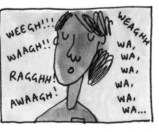

A nurse tells me I need to spend a night sleeping by James on the baby unit to get used to him. 'I think you should stay tonight.'

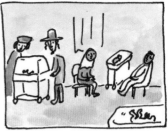

Other anxious parents all doing the same thing. We all try to give each other space, quietly talking or singing to our babies. So unlike being at home.

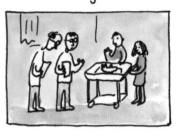

Overhear a lot of conversations about feeding tubes. 'But if you took it out she might learn to drink by herself and we could take her home.' 'Sorry, can't take it out till she's strong enough.'

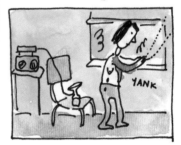

I like having the curtains open.

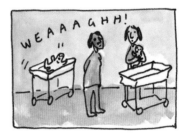

'Right. OK.' Seems more like I'll be 'getting used to' the other baby, but I agree to it.

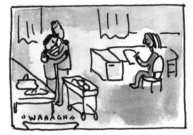

There's a neat fold-out bed
by his tray.
'Night, baby, see you and
James in the morning.'
'Night night.'

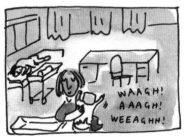

Get more sleep than I expected.
Night nurse soothes the big
baby and I wear earplugs.
(Not what I'd do at home.)

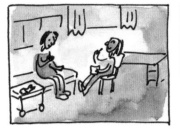

Hungry after feeding James
at 4am. Share my pretzel
sticks with the nurse.
She tells me everyone in
Colombia has annual CT Scans
to catch cancer early.
If only I'd done that!
'Take these away from me,
I'll eat the lot!.'

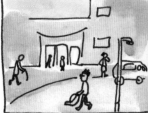

After 10 days we can
take James home.
Mum brings the
baby seat.

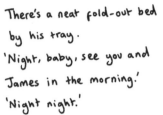

He's too tiny for it and
flops over to one side.

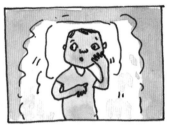

Back at home, he looks
a bit discombobulated.

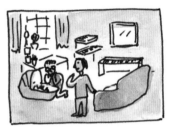

'Wow, we've got a baby
in the house... what shall
we do now?'
'I'm just going to sit here
and worship him for a bit.'

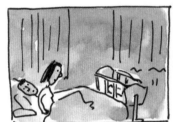

He sleeps well the first night.
Me and Tom both wake up
every time he moves.
'What's he doing?
Is he breathing OK?'

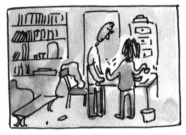

Working out how to change
his nappy.
'How is one person meant to
do this??'
'Argh, he weed in his face,
pass me that...'

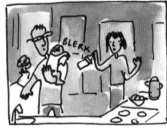

Now he's home he really is
a great distraction.
'Is this stuff sterile?'
'Oh gawd, I dunno.'
'Oop, he's been sick again.'

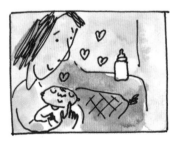

Sometimes I forget
what I'm anxious about.

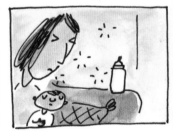

Then remember again.

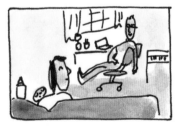

Wonder about simple things.
'How are you supposed to
do stuff like go to the shop?'
'I dunno, let's think about
it tomorrow.'

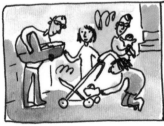

Tom's mum and sister come
and help us put the
pram together.
'I put two nappies in,
you think that'll
be enough?'

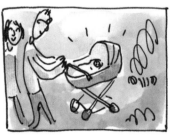

Take James on his first
trip to the park.
He seems even tinier outside.

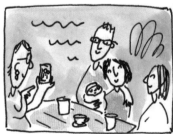

'That's a lovely pic!.'

JULY

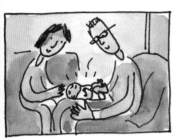

We spend a lot of time just staring at him and waiting to see what he does.

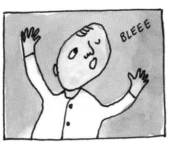

When he's hungry he bleats like a little goat.

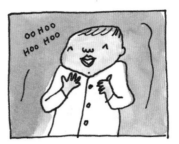

When he's falling asleep he chirrups and looks like he's remembering an old joke from ages ago.

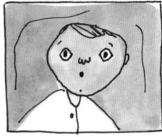

Sometimes he just stares at you like it's the end of the universe.

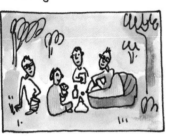

Another trip to the park with our friends Matt and Matt (we know a lot of Matts). Have fun playing a game guessing how much tickets to Glastonbury cost in different years.

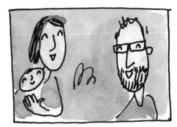

'1999?'
'Mm... £80?'

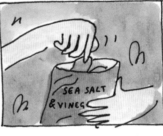

'Yes! £83.'
'Hehe.'
'Think I did a whitey in a ditch that year.'

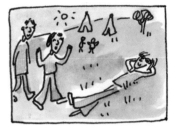

That was the year I bumped into Tom, before I knew him very well, lying on the grass in the teepee field. Imagine if we'd known about all this!

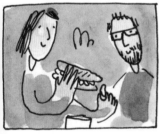

I make a cheese and crisp sandwich. Matt says how well I'm dealing with things. 'I'm such a softie, I don't know how I'd cope!'

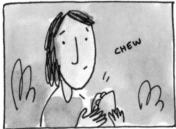

I feel like I'm coping well on the outside.

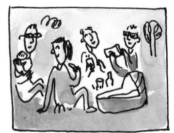

Also like I'm on the edge of breaking down, most of the time.

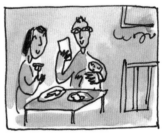

'1995?'
'Hmm, I think I jumped the fence that year.'
'Only £65! £205 now, what a rip-off.'

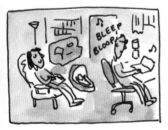

Peaceful evening, me drawing, Tom listening to Raymond Scott, baby on the floor between us.
'You think he likes this?'

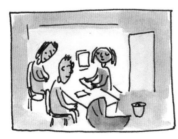

The next morning, we go to register the baby at Hackney town hall.
'Is it Tom or Thomas?'
'Thomas.'
'Occupation please?'
'Childminder.'

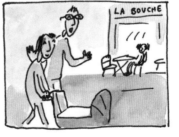

'Damn, I should've said I'm something cooler. I should've said I'm an "ENTREPRENEUR", a childminding entrepreneur!'

Have banana pancakes to celebrate James being an official human. There's something on the menu called 'Snazzy beans'. 'Damn, should've called him that! Little Snazzy Bean!'

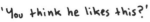

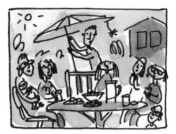

Take James for his first trip out of Hackney for breakfast in Polly's garden.
'Not that umbrella, Felix! It's too spidery!'
'I thought you wanted shade!?'
'No no, I don't, I don't!'

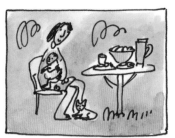

At one point I have a newborn baby in my arms and their new kitten, Ishmail, curled up on my feet. Cute!

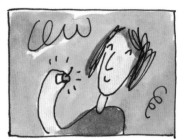

Eat small orange cherries from their tree and talk about how good it is that people are taking an interest in my work since I've been writing this comic.

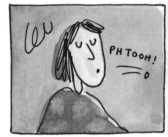

'I will have to start giving uplifting speeches about how getting cancer was the best thing I ever did.'

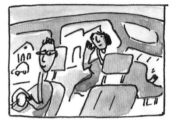

On the way back I get nostalgic driving past the warehouses I used to live in.
'I miss those margarine tubs used as ash trays.'
(Still with marge in.)
'And the trapeze artists.'
My old life seems so far away.

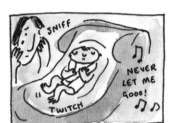

Now ALL music on the radio makes me cry.
'James can't get enough of the autotune!
Can't believe this junk has set me off.'

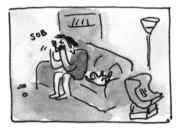

Our flat is full of assorted baby seats. The one from the car can also be used as a rocker.
'Can't get the bottom bit off.'
'Try pressing the grey things.'
'I AM pressing the grey things, it's not working!'

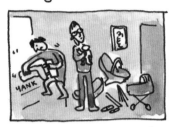

'Fucking baby seats!'
I feel a complete mess.

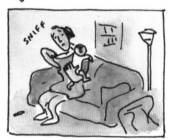

Crying all the time, covered in baby sick, wondering if it's me or him that smells of shit.

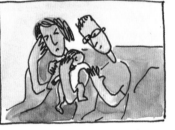

'I'm a terrible girlfriend and mother, so unfun, might die...'
'No you're not, me and Jim are lucky to have you.'

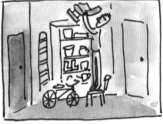

Tom finds a place for one of the baby seats in the hall.
'Might be useful when he's a bit bigger.'

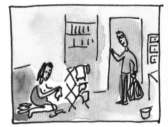

We tidy up the flat together and I feel a bit better.
'That's more like it.'

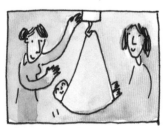

Next day some sweet midwives come to weigh James.
'Nearly 7Lbs, very good boy.'

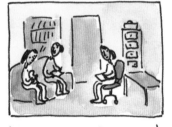

'Now, are you feeling stressed or anxious at all?'
'Well, er, yes, but Tom and Mum are helping.'
'Lovely.'

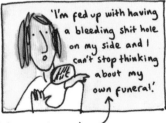

I bet if I said

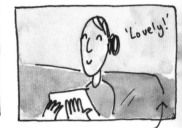

They would still say

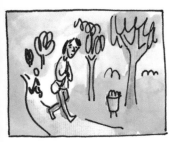

Know I'm feeling more anxious at the moment because I've got to have a CT scan to see if there's been any cancer recurrence. Walk to hospital through the park.

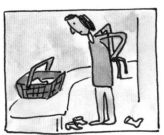

Own clothes go in a red plastic shopping basket. Hospital gown is quite hard to do up at the back.

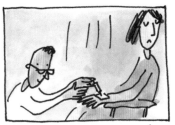

I still hate having blood tests and cannulas put in. 'Not a fan of needles?' 'Nope, still can't look after all this time.'

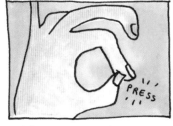

I have a trick to distract myself: I dig my thumbnail into my finger so it hurts more than the needle going in.

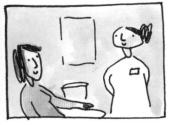

The radiographer remembers me from my first CT scan on the day of my diagnosis in February. 'You're looking much better! It's nice to see people doing well.' 'Yes, and the baby is fine.'

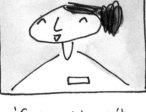

'Fantastic! I wasn't going to ask.'

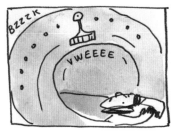

I don't remember the CT scanner sounding like a washing machine, or the cycloptic light, or having to put my arms above my head.

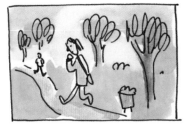

Buy a hot cross bun as a treat for the way home. Will get scan results in a couple of days.

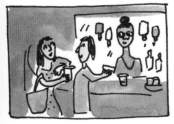

That evening I leave James with Tom and go for a Campari cocktail on the roof of some studios with my friend Emer.

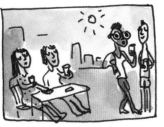

It's nice to have the sun beaming right into my face. Emer tells me about the Venice Biennale. 'We were trying to do this sound installation thing in a basement but we kept getting kicked out.'

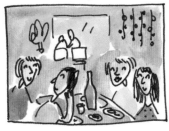

Then meet our friends Lily and Nell for Vietnamese food on Kingsland Road. 'He was quite fit. Funny teeth, though.'

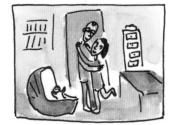

'Ah, my boys! I had a normal night out, it was great!'

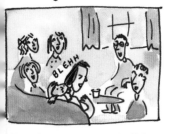

Day before scan results. Lots of friends come to meet James. He puts on a good show and is sick in my face.

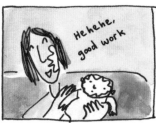

We look like we've been hit with custard pies.

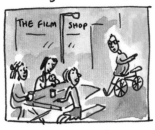

Go and sit outside a bar and have some waters. My friend Finn just avoids having his bike nicked. 'You ran so fast!' 'He just said "oh sorry, is it yours?", wish I'd said something hard and cool.'

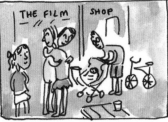

Everyone wishes me love and luck. 'Bye, dude, love you, amazing person.' 'Bye, little Jedi, nice to meet you.' (James looks like a Jedi wrapped in his pale brown blanket.)

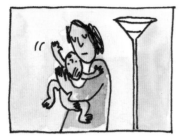

Give baby one last hug before I go to appt with oncologist. He's hungry and doesn't want to be hugged. Mum will meet me at hospital with him later.

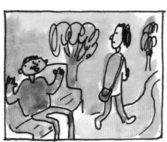

Bloke talking to himself tells me I've got a 'NICE BUM!' Well, if one good thing happens today...

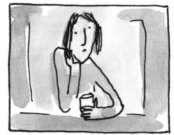

Blood tests out of the way quickly - have a couple of hours to kill and go to a cafe. Keep forgetting to breathe properly.

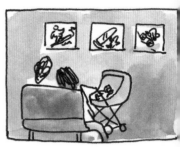

Find Mum and James in outpatients waiting room. James makes a tiny noise.

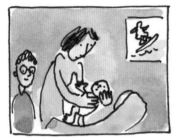

'Think he needs comforting.' Me that needs comforting.

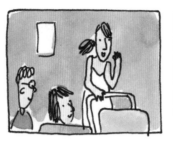

Oncologist coos over the baby. I think, 'She wouldn't be doing that if it were bad news'. 'Oh bless him, so gorgeous!'

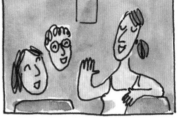

'Well, you're all clear, nothing exciting on your scans at all.' 'Oh phew! What a relief!' 'Wonderful!'

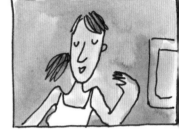

'Apart from a residual fecal mass.'

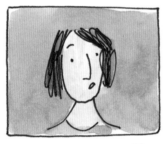

'What does that mean?'

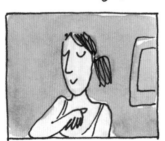

'That you needed the toilet.'

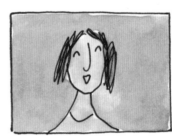

'Oh yes, so I did.'

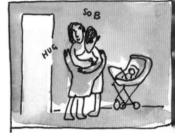

Outside the consulting room. 'Well done, darling. You were worried, weren't you?' 'Yes, but I wasn't letting myself be as worried as I actually was.' 'I know.'

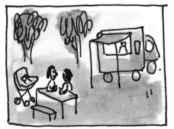

Have a roast veg focaccia at a cafe in the park to celebrate. Clear scan means carrying on with the next 3 months of chemo as planned, as it's probably doing its job.

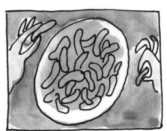

Extra plate of gherkins on the side. 'PHEW! I can relax for another few months.' (Next scan.) 'Hmm, I never really liked gherkins...'

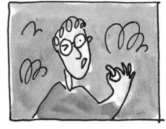

'Nope, still don't. Blech! So pointless.'

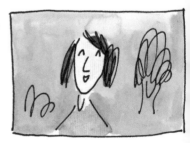

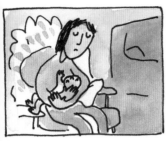

Sad to have to stop breastfeeding. (Chemo starts again in a few days.)

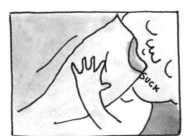

Enjoy a couple of good feeds before cutting down.

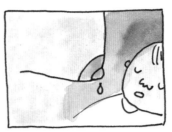

Feels all wrong to poison something so amazing and natural.

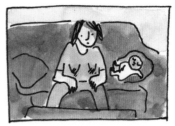

Tits leak for days.

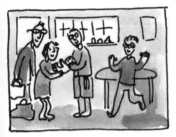

Take James home to Sussex for the first time. 'Can you hold him for a min?' 'Hello, little James!'

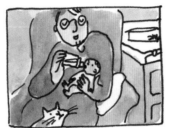

Mikey feeds him while we bring stuff in from the car. The cat looks put out.

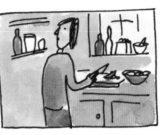

Make a salad for me and Tom. 'Burp him properly or he'll be sick!'

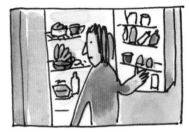

I feel agitated... 'Where are the pine nuts??'

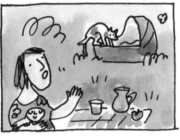

And overprotective. 'No, cat! Not in there!'

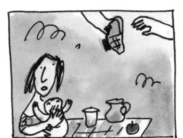

'Dog poo, sorry, must've picked it up in the lane.' 'Oh dear, let me deal with that.' 'Take it away!!'

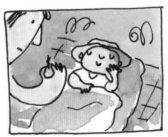

'Ant! Get off my baby!'

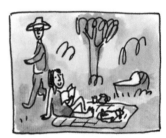

Relax, eventually. 'Just going for a walk, you be alright here for a bit?' 'Mmhm.'

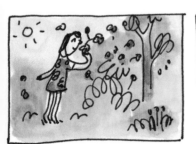

Wander about the garden with bare feet, while the baby sleeps, sniffing roses and stuff.

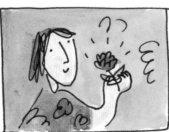

Pick a really nice one and think about putting it in my hair.

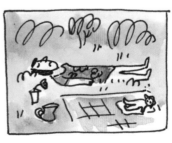

Then remember my horrible ruined body and put it in a glass instead.

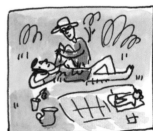

'Nice walk?' 'Yeh, only saw two people.'

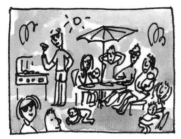

BBQ with old school friends. We talk about people we used to know.
'First pair of boobs I ever saw.'

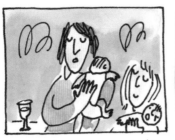

Conversations about feeding babies etc.
'I don't know <u>how</u> women manage breastfeeding on their own.'
'Oh, you just manage.'

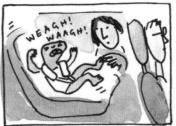

Traffic jam on the way back to London.
'Poor little frog, too hot, isn't it?'

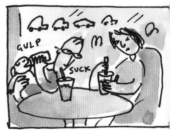

Cry into a frappuccino at Starbucks on the M23.
'I don't know who I am any more, I'm just a cancer baby person.'

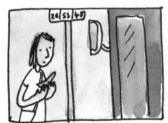

Feel a bit better talking to a man in the carpark about how cute James is.
'He's not even meant to be born yet!' 'Ah, lovely!'
(The man was just trying to get to his car but was too polite to say so.)

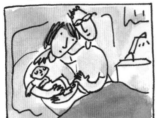

Back at home.
'Sorry I keep having a meltdown the whole time.'
'That's OK. Sorry I don't know what to say when you have a meltdown.'

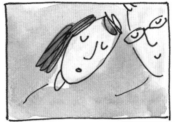

'Oh just the usual stuff is fine, just tell me I'm great and you love me and it'll all be alright and things...'

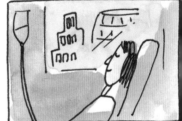

'You ARE great and I love you and I'm sure it's all gone.'

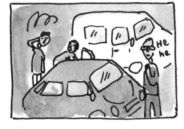

First day back at chemo, waiting for the bus. Feels like going back to school in September used to. Have sharpened my pencils and bought a banana.

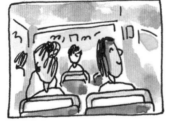

Whenever I'm having crap times in the summer I think of Bergman's film Summer with Monika. Then I remember when Tom called it Monika's Shitty Holiday and it makes me laugh.

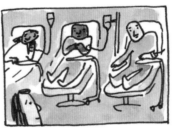

My chair is in the treatment room without any windows. Three fed-up old people all staring at me. Not one of them moves or says 'hello'. I feel like I'm watching Waiting for Godot.

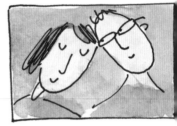

Nurses let me move to a room with a window. It means I have a normal chair instead of a comfy treatment chair but I don't mind at all.

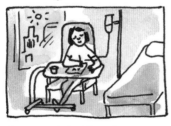

I appreciate the air-con and get on with some work. Could almost imagine I'm 'hot-desking' in a trendy office.

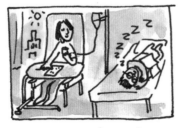

Mum arrives and immediately falls asleep on the bed next to me. Gentle snoring. Slightly less like hot-desking.

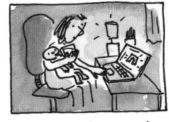

Up late, wired on steroids. Quite good for night-time feeds. Unintentional shopping bender: Handbag, trousers, flip-flops, weird silver shoes, electric fan.

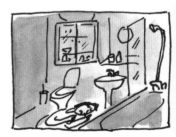

Then suddenly feel sick and exhausted and have to lie down on the bathroom floor. Should've tried to go to bed earlier.

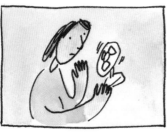

The fan I bought online arrives. It's titchy.
'Not much good, they all looked big on the website!'

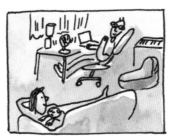

All still boiling. Shelter from the sun with the curtains closed and the titchy fan on.
'Think it just blew your fart across the room.'
'At least it's good for something.'

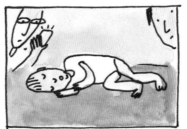

Baby's floppy in the heat.
'Do you think we should give him water?'
'Internet says "no".'

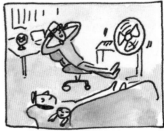

Polly lends us a giant fan.
'Ahh, much better, just like having a Christmas tree in the room.'

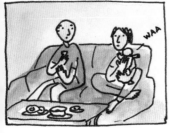

Alan comes to visit after a heavy night out.
We eat bagels and hummus.
'I don't believe in babies.'
'Hm, well, I'm afraid he's real!'

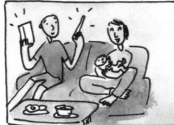

'Anyway, I need you to take photos of me in the park making giant bubbles with this thing I got. James will shit himself over it.'
'Of course!'

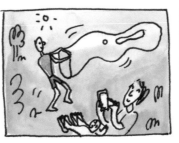

'Wooooh, great one!'
'Hey, now we're weird hippie people with a bubble thing and a baby in the park!'

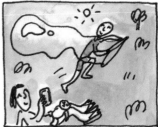

'And you're wearing flip-flops, argh!'
'Haha, I love these flip-flops!'
Normal with each other again.

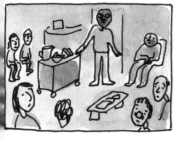

Go to get my dressing changed. No one reacts at all when the refreshments man comes and says, 'Tea? Coffee? Sandwich please?'

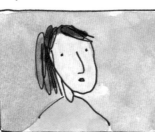

He looks a bit annoyed and I say, 'I'm fine, thanks,' loudly.

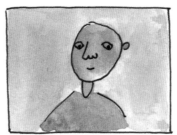

He looks a bit less annoyed.

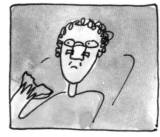

Woman without a nose already has her own sandwich.

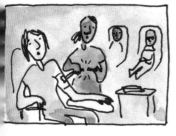

My PICC line breaks as the nurse is changing the bandage.
'Oh no! Wait there, Matilda, don't touch anything.'

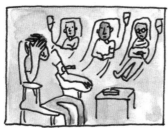

Start to cry because I think they'll have to put the whole thing in again. More staring old blokes.

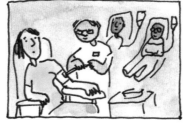

Brilliant nurse manages to fix it and talks to me soothingly about fans.
'I don't know whether to get the metal or plastic kind.'
One of the old blokes says, 'You were lucky.' I was.

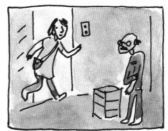

Run and jump into the lift just as doors are closing.
Smile at the porter.
'Can't get out of here fast enough, eh?'
'Yup.'

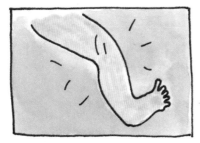

Baby is growing into his skin already. I miss those baggy knees!

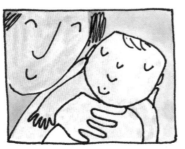

He's getting a good double chin, too. I feel proud of it!

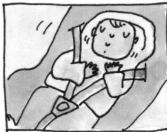

His cheeks judder when I'm pushing him around in his pushchair.

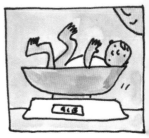

He weighs nearly 9lbs now, almost twice his birth weight, in 6 weeks!

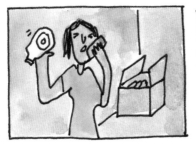

Having a nightmare with the colostomy bag suppliers. 'You sent me the wrong kind AGAIN! Now I've got to spend ANOTHER day at home waiting for them to be delivered!'

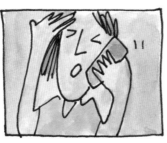

They ask why I want to order more this time. 'Why do you THINK? It's not as if I WANT hundreds of colostomy bags cluttering up my flat?! What else am I going to use them for other than to collect my own shit???'

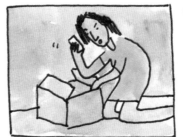

They always send lots of deliveries of small things in big boxes... 'Just some adhesive remover, in this big box?! They must be taking the piss.'

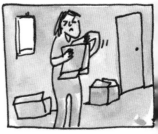

...which means our hall is always full of boxes. I HATE COLLAPSING BOXES!

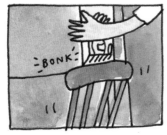

Also annoyed with our tiny kitchen. The fridge door bashes the chair every time you open it.

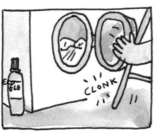

The washing machine door bashes the chair on the other side.

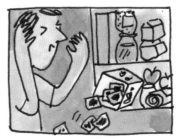

Not enough room on the shelves. Knock a load of teabags on the floor. 'AAAAAARRRGHH!!!!'

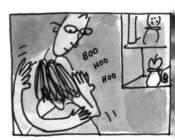

Tom hears me roaring from the other room. 'What is it? What happened??' 'Knocked some teabags on the floor.' 'Oh dear.'

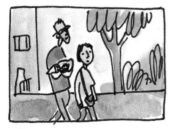

That evening we take James for a walk round the block to settle him. 'Ah, it's good to get outside.'

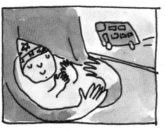

He likes hearing buses going by. I agree, they almost sound like waves.

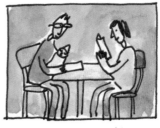

We sit outside the Georgian cafe. 'Think I'll have bean stew tonight.'

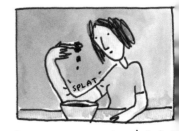

It tastes very nice but is a bit brown and gloopy. 'Trust me to order a bowl of shit for dinner.'

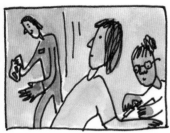

Go for another blood test. Man whose job it is to collect samples has a dodgy bowl cut, very long nails and black fingerless gloves. He really looks the part.

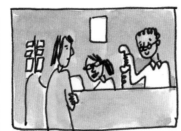

Handing my blood test in to be sent away for genetic analysis. Am annoyed with the receptionists, flirting and taking ages over it. 'You phone them.' 'No you phone them.' (HURRY UP SO I CAN GET THE FUCK OUT OF HERE.)

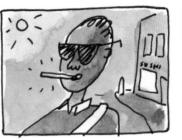

Other interesting people I notice that day: A man in aviators looking cool chewing a biro.

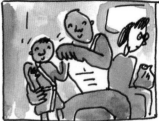

A little boy in a judo kit on the bus, inventing jokes that don't make sense. 'How can a chicken drink? Chicken wing fingers!' Muscle twat dad pretends to punch him in the face.

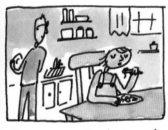

One evening, the little girl Tom looks after suddenly says: 'Matty started chemo again.'

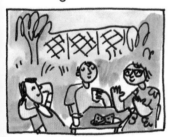

Tom hadn't mentioned it to her, he laughs.

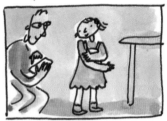

'Well don't laugh! It's not going to make her feel very nice!'

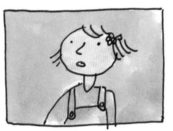

Tom texts to say she wants to tell me she's been bitten by a mosquito. (He told her I had been bitten by one too, the night before.) 'Matty says we should squash all those guys!' 'Yes, but not the beetles.'

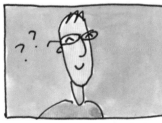

Go to Lucy's to do some singing with Polly. Tea and watermelon in the sun first. Her garden is lovely and overgrown. Talk about the Royal Baby. 'So lucky he's not a James!'

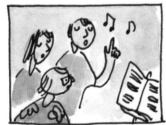

Manage to sing without crying (result!). Georgian, Yiddish, Spanish and Japanese folk songs. It's good to do some sight-reading and exercise my brain.

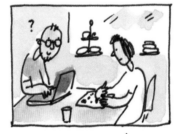

Next day, my blood count is too low to have chemo so me and Mikey have a long working lunch. 'I might have a
*   *   *   *
    lager shandy.
*   *   *   *
fancy one?' 'Nah, better stick to water.'

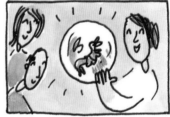

My aunt and uncle, Tom + Jill, come to visit. They bring the plate from Nan's house that looks like a rabbit with its bum showing. 'Thank you!'

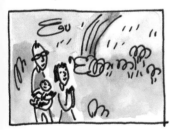

Take James to Sussex again. There's a BEAUTIFUL rainbow over the fields. 'Oh! So mind-blowing!' (James not that interested.)

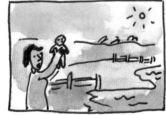

Take him to see the sea... 'Look, James! The Channel! The curve of the earth!'

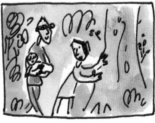

...for a walk in the woods... 'Such a huge tree! It grew from nothing, just like you, laddie.'

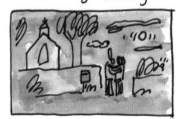

...and to see the sun set at my favourite spot by the church. 'Maybe you'll be a sun worshipper like me, James.' 'Hehe, I love it when you're being cosmic.'

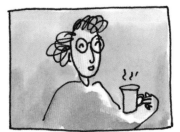

Another thing I want to add, and there's no good place for it really, is that I HATE hearing about other people's cancer experiences:
'Of course when Roger died, bla bla bla...'

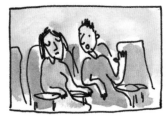

'And do you have to pay for parking at hospital?'
'Yup.'
'We did too, so annoying.'

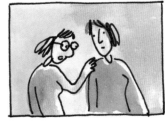

I guess if people's relatives have died of cancer they <u>do</u> need to talk about it.

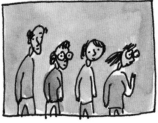

So as to avoid:
'Do you always have to wait this long?'
'Yup.'

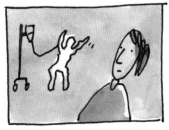

Especially if they died. I feel like I'm being chased by ghosts.

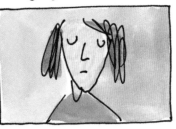

The whole thing is so ÜBER FUCKING ANNOYING.
I don't feel like complaining about the tiny things. It makes it all seem worse. (Also I feel lucky to be being treated for free etc etc etc.)

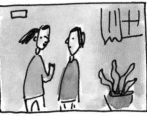

But I am definitely not the right person to talk about it with.

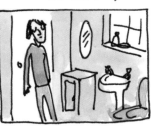

And: 'So why do you need another blood test, then?'
'Ahm, I have one every time, to see if I can have chemo or not.'

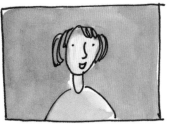

'It was really amazing, my Mum lived for 12 years after her diagnosis!'

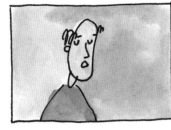

'Judy looked like a skeleton at first.'
Sometimes it's as if people want to show they aren't afraid to talk about it.

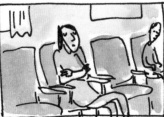

Sometimes I prefer going to hospital on my own so I don't have to explain what's happening to anyone.

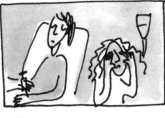

Talking about those things reminds me what a pain it all is.
'Eek, how horrible, I hate needles.'
'Me too.'

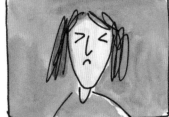

That's not amazing. That's shit!
I want to live for another 50 at least! None of these people relate to me. So I don't want to know.

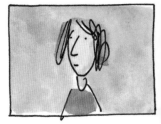

'Um, I've just got to go to the loo.'
Best thing to do is walk away. They're only trying to be nice.

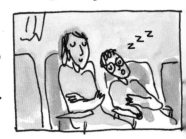

Or with people who I don't have to explain anything to.

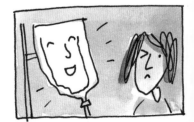

I also hate it when people say 'chemo' (although I say it). It's such a friendly sounding abbreviation. I prefer saying 'treatment'. Silly, I know.

AUGUST

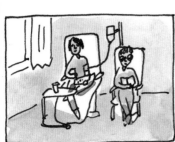

Next dose of chemo is uneventful.

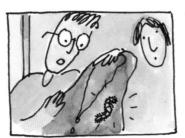

Apart from Mum finding a centipede on her jacket at the bus stop on the way home.

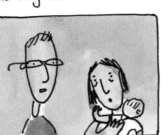

She flicks it off.

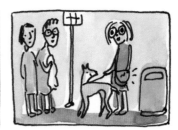

It lands on the bag of a cross woman with a greyhound.
'Whoops, sorry.'
'Get rid of it, please!'
(I flick it off her bag.)

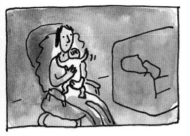

Up all night, wired on steroids.
Baby won't settle.

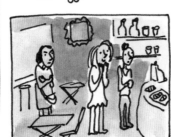

'How was he?'
'Oh, annoying.'
'Sorry I didn't wake up.'
'I was awake anyway so don't worry about it.'
Steroids make me snappy and aggravated.

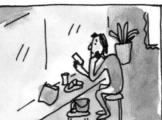

More thrashing and grunting.
'Stupid baby.'

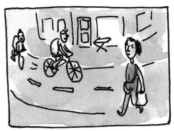

Go out to the post office, feel angry...
'All these pricks in linen shirts on nice bikes looking happy and not having cancer.'

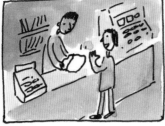

... then elated and madly over-friendly...
Post office man manages to pack my large package into a small envelope.
'WE DID IT! WOOHOO!'

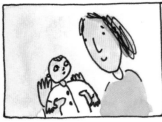

People keep asking if James is smiling yet.
'Come on little boglin, smile for Mummy...'

... then angry again...
Stop for a croissant on the way home.
'Ooh, these all look so yummy, I just don't know which one to have!'
'They're only croissants for fuck's sake, just choose one' (thinks).

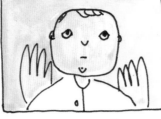

He isn't, really.

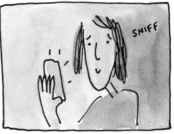

... then guilty about calling James a 'stupid baby'...
Text Tom to say sorry and to tell him I've bought him a croissant.

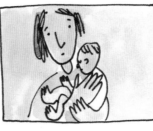

At 9 weeks old, I can see they're thinking
'AUTISM???'
when they ask.
I guess he hasn't had much to smile about.

... then weepy and emotional...
Tom texts back to say don't worry, sometimes he calls James similar things, and that he's just eaten a flat old croissant he found in my bag.
'I love those guys so much!'
Steroid mood swings.

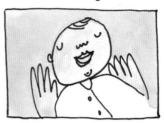

Sometimes he smiles in his sleep. I wonder if that counts.

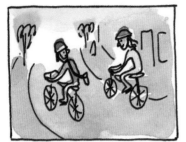

Ride to the cinema with Claire. First time I've cycled since January. 'What a rush, I'm a happy prick on a bike!'

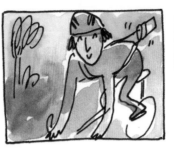

Chemo pump bouncing in the breeze. 'Almost as carefree as an open linen shirt!'

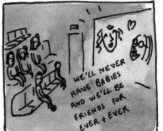

We meet Cesca and go to see the film Frances Ha.

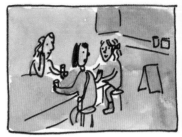

'They just went on about what great friends they were without actually having a very good friendship at all!'

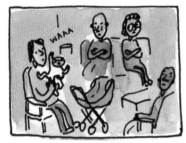

Take James with me to have chemo pump unplugged. Bit of a mistake.

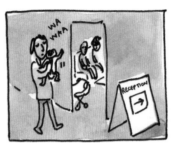

Chemo ward is no place for a baby, really. 'Shh, it's OK, laddie, we'll be out of here soon.'

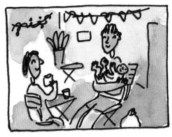

Meet my friend Rob for a cup of tea at the city farm on our way back. 'What a peachy little dude!' 'Hehe, babies suit you! You should get one too!'

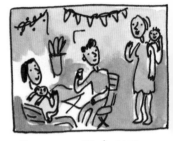

Strangers with babies often stop to chat. '2 months? What a sweetheart. And how are you coping?' 'Oh, fine, great!'

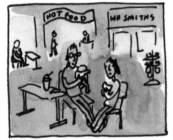

Drive to Nottingham for the weekend. Stop at Northampton services and talk about the big things. 'I certainly don't believe in that kind of God, but I can't help feeling cosmic about some stuff.'

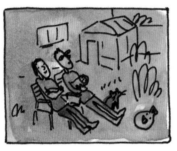

That night, we sit in the garden, looking for Perseids (meteors). 'Come on, God, gimme everything you've got.'

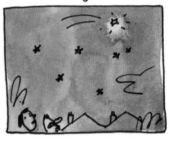

'There's one, look!' We see 3 before it gets a bit cold.

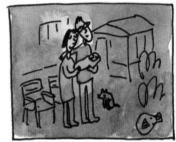

'Shall we go in? My neck hurts.' 'Yeh.' 'Ahh, love you guys.'

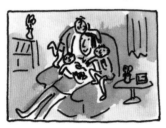

Catch nits off the nephews. 'You can hold him in a minute.'

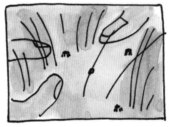

Looking for nits. 'Aargh. This is the last thing we need.'

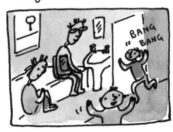

Hide in the bathroom with nit stuff in our hair. 'Uncle Tom! Uncle Tom!' 'You can't come in, we're covered in chemicals.' 'How long do we leave it on?' '15 mins.' 'Maybe we could stay in here for 20...'

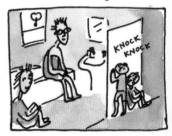

'Just like hiding in the bathroom at a party. All I need is a roll-up and a warm tin of Tyskie.' 'Hehe.'

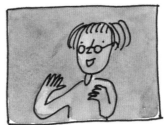

Just remembered another thing I hate, that I forgot to mention earlier: When people tell me about the time they thought they had cancer...
'All this blood in my poo...'

'...weird lump in my neck...'

'...an abnormal smear test...'

'... something itchy on my hand...'

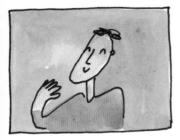

...but it turns out that they didn't. 'It was only piles.'

'...just an infection.'

'... nothing serious.'

'...only a mole!'
<u>LUCKY YOU.</u>

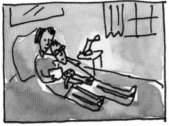

Tom is usually unbelievably calm. (Asleep with baby.)

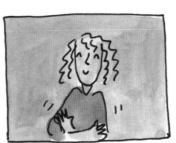

One evening he wakes up with a start.

'You alright?'

'Just feeling panicked. I often wake up feeling panicked.' I never knew.

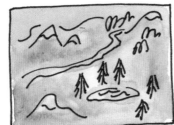

'Let's go away somewhere when this is all over.' We look at bits of Scotland on the iPad.

'Hey, there's a place called Keith!'

'I really want to go to Aberdeen and see what effect all that North Sea oil has had on it.'

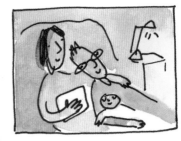

'What will we do when I don't have to go to hospital any more?'
'Worry about all the stuff we used to worry about, I guess.'

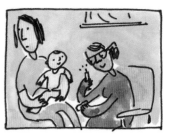

Take James to be immunised, he's in quite a good mood.
'Hold his leg still while I do the injection.'

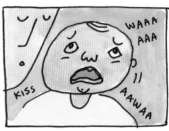

He looks bewildered and screams his head off when she does it.
'What a brave boy.'

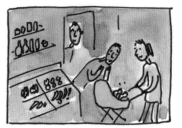

He calms down quite quickly and we go to the veg shop. Love how unguardedly broody the shop blokes are.
'Ahh, so little, what is he thinking, I wonder?'

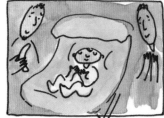

Man buying a banana joins in too.
'So adorable, that thing they do with their hands!'

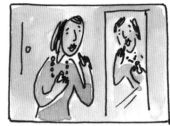

Leave James with Claire and cycle to hospital to get my dressing changed. Feel invincible, cycling for cancer treatment!

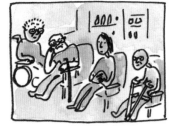

Everyone in the waiting room seems even older than usual. Funny, sitting with my bike helmet next to them with their sticks and wheelchairs.

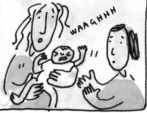

Get home and Claire's looking stressed. James has been screaming for hours.
'Did I do something wrong?'
'Ohh, I'm sorry! It's fine, it might be the jabs.'

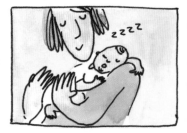

Eventually he calms down and has a good sleep on my shoulder.
'That's a bit better.'

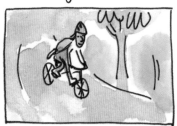

Friday evening, I get ready to go to my friend Amy's hen party. Put on some makeup for the first time in months.
'I look quite good!'

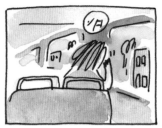

Suddenly cry on the bus, I think, because putting on makeup and going out for the evening is normal and fun, and it feels good to be doing normal, fun things again.

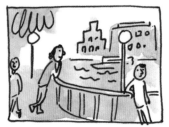

Arrive a bit early and go for a walk along the South Bank. Spend a while taking it all in.

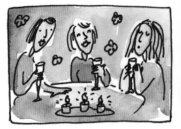

The hen party is very civilised (I'm missing the clubbing trip). We talk about hen-party-type things.
'I'm sorry, but it's just not possible to be friends with your boyfriend's ex.'
'So, are you married?'
'Nope.'

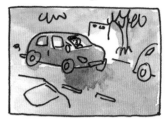

Saturday evening, I drive to Matt and Ruth's in Barnet for Matt's birthday party. Feel excited to be driving. Try a new route via Palmer's Green and manage without looking at a map. (I am a real route nerd.)

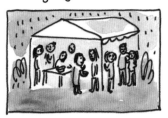

Stand around eating chickpea salad.
'How's the wee one?'
'He's fine, really big! Startles himself every time he makes a noise.'
'Hehe, excellent.'

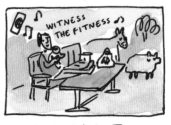

On Sunday I take James to Spitalfields city farm. Pigs and a donkey walk by. I buy a bag of kale.
'This is hiphop, James, what do you think?'

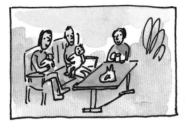

Meet my friends Cathy + Brendan and their son, Aidan. Talk about Brendan's dad, who died of bowel cancer earlier in the year. (I started the conversation so I don't mind.)

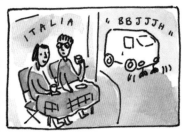

Before next chemo, me and Mum have coffee at an Italian cafe. She tells me I should do pelvic floor exercises. A very loud street cleaner drives by and she has to shout: 'So that your...

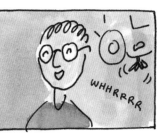

...BUM HOLE STILL WORKS.'

(When I have the operation reversed.)

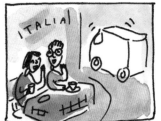

It keeps driving back and forth for ages right by us. We get the giggles and have fun shouting 'BUM HOLE' over the sound of the engine.

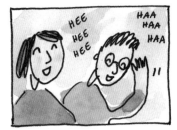

Hysterics.

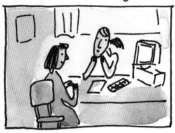

Appointment with oncologist to go through my symptoms from the last dose. Tell her I've been getting pins and needles in my feet. 'Ah. How badly?' 'Mm, I don't know, badlyish?'

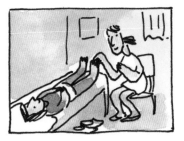

She gets me to take my shoes off and does a test with a drawing-pin-type thing to see if I can feel it poking my toes or not. 'Yep, feels sharp.'

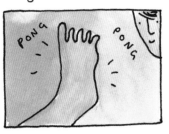

'You didn't think you were going to have to take your shoes off today, did you!' 'Nope!'

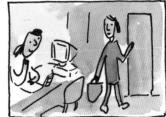

'Just let me know if it gets any worse, could be permanent nerve damage. Otherwise see you in a month and it'll be nearly over!' 'See you then!' 'Bye now.'

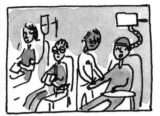

Another uneventful dose. Cheerful woman with a loud laugh next to me. 'Can you use my other arm? My veins get harder every time, AHAHAHA!'

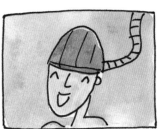

She's wearing a cold cap so her hair stays on. 'I'm a bit of a pin cushion to tell you the truth!!!!!'

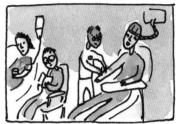

'WOOHOO, you got it in! You must be some sort of vein magician, AHAHAHAHAHH!'

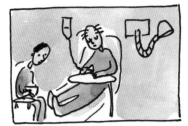

Later on, she's talking to her husband with the cap off. She's almost completely bald and I wonder why she's bothering with it. 'It's just rather a long time to wait for a sandwich, that's all.'

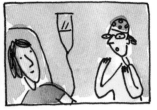

I offer to show my PICC line to another woman who's freaking out about getting hers. 'Oh gawd, did it hurt?'

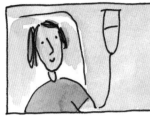

'A little bit, but they were very gentle with it all.'

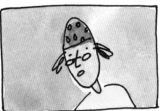

She wants to complain. 'I think they could be a bit more sympathetic. When I had cancer 17 years ago, a nurse would sit and talk to you for hours. Don't get nothing like that now.'

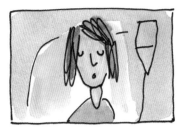

'Well I think they do a very good job.'

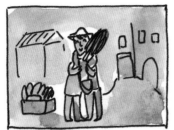

The next day I meet up with Leigh, a friend of a friend. She's being treated for Hodgkin's Lymphoma at the same hospital as me. We've been emailing a bit and give each other a huge hug. 'Ahh, hello!'

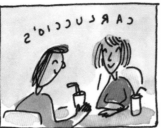

I had thought I didn't want to make any cancer mates, but it's actually really good to talk to someone who knows what it's like. 'Had to have this needle stuck in my chest, I felt like a burger on a spike.' 'Argh, so horrible!'

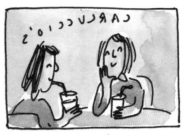

We chat for hours. 'I can't stand it when people try to do things for me like washing up, I feel so out of control.' 'Oh really? I love it when people turn up and do the cleaning!' ←(me)

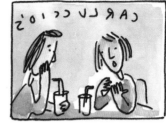

Comparing tumours. 'Big ones by my heart and lungs.' 'Could you feel them?' 'Not at all, doctor said it was asthma.' 'Awful!'

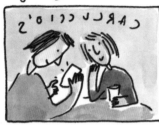

Arrange to do a cancer patients make-over day together. 'Would it be awful?' 'It might be funny!' 'Yeah, let's do it!'

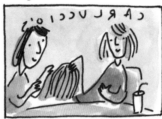

She picked up a wig that morning. 'Want to see?' 'But your hair looks fine!' 'It's all falling out!' 'You can't tell at all.'

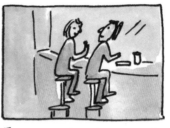

Then we go to get some sushi and talk about other stuff. It's nice to have things in common that aren't cancer. 'Oh I love Bruce Lacey's films, so playful!' (video art)

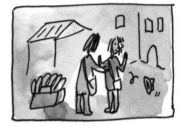

'Was really great to meet up!' 'Whoops, knocked your hat off.' 'Hope you feel ok this week.' 'You too.'

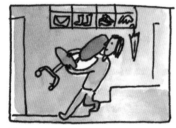

Pumped on steroid energy, I finally get rid of my horrible old broken office chair. 'At last.'

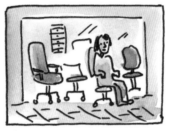

Go and try out other horrible office chairs in the second-hand furniture shop down the road. Try to find the least horrible one.

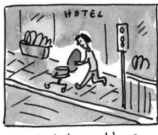

Wheel it home. I have a mad idea about reupholstering it with a cool old jumper.

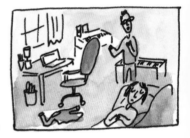

More difficult than I thought. 'It's huge!' 'I know, I think I hate it even more than the old one.' 'Ah well, at least it'll be comfy.'

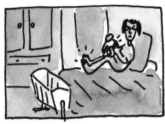

Side effects are quite bad this time. Feet are burning and my hands hurt too much to burp the baby. 'Oh fucking hell.'

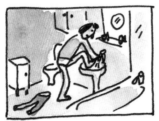

Tom heats us up some pies and I run my feet under the cold tap.

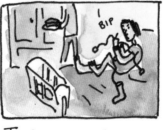

Try to figure out an electronic pain relief thing that me and Mum bought on the internet a while ago.

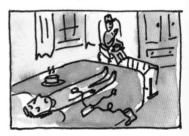

Can't be arsed with it.

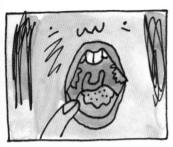

Get loads of mouth ulcers.
Back of my throat is raw.

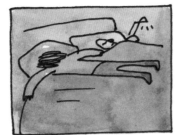

Body aches all over,
it's as if I've got
too much blood.

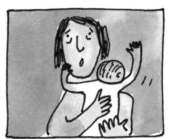

Finally get to sleep then
baby wakes up and needs
feeding. Feel totally ragged.

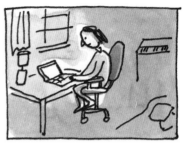

Later in the week,
I manage to send 2 emails.
Zenith of productivity.

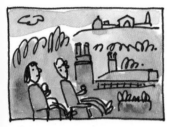

Side-effects wear off a
bit by the weekend and
we go to house-sit at Polly's.
It's lovely sitting on their
roof terrace looking at
Alexandra Palace.
'So wish we had a
house like this.'
'Love being up in the trees.'

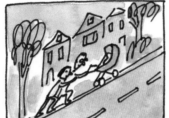

Go on an outing to
Muswell Hill.
'Forgot what a steep
climb it is.'

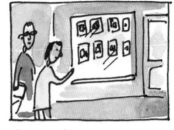

Look in the windows of an
estate agent and pretend
we can afford the houses.
'That one's perfect! 3 bed,
garden and terrace, only
1 and a bit million.'
'Let's get it!'

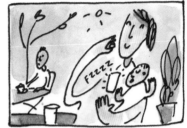

Stop at a child-friendly cafe.
White noise app on my phone
by the baby's head so he sleeps,
drop sourdough crumbs all
over him.
'Ha ha, we've become
✳ THOSE PEOPLE ✳'

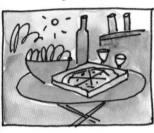

Later, we get takeaway
pizza to have while
we watch the sunset
over the rooves.

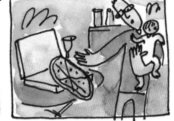

Tom accidentally knocks
it off the table...

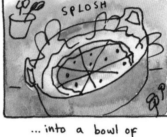

...into a bowl of
dirty old water.

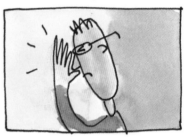

'FUUCKK, NOOOO!'
I don't think I've ever
seen him look more upset.

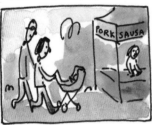

Take James to a farmers'
market.
'What you gonna get?'
'Coffee, and some sort of
bun-type-thing.'
'Think I want a smoothie.'
'James, your mother is
making me look bad.'

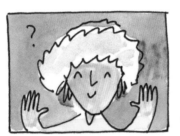

'Shall I buy an
alpaca fur hat?'
Not this time.

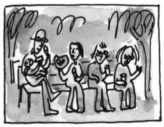

We eat ice creams on a bench.
'Guy gave me a free pretzel!'
Woman next to us is boring
her friend with a dreary
monologue.
'It's just I'm a burden,
I know I am... still, I met
up with my cousin who is
just lovely, except of course
she's got lung cancer...

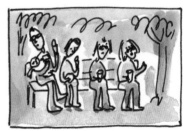

...She really hasn't got long.
Anyway, I was thinking
I could take you out for
dinner tonight with a few
of your friends, or maybe
just me and you?'
Cancer following me
around again.

SEPTEMBER

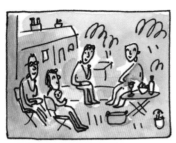

Dinner on the roof with Adam + Alan. We talk about looking after children.
'Had to take my nephews to Go Ape, it was a fucking nightmare!'

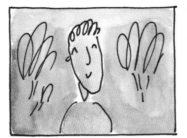

'The 12-year-old kept pushing me off the rope walk.'
'Ha! Miserable.'
'I just feel like a big child around the kids in my family...'

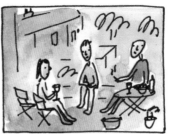

Tom puts James to bed and we talk about how I like to keep cancer life separate from social life.
'You know we'd come with you to hospital if you wanted us to...'
'It's what friends are for!'

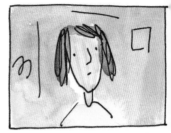

'I know, it's just I don't really want any of my friends to see me like that, hooked up to drips looking sad. They might be upset. Or I guess I would be upset.'

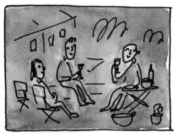

Stay outside talking and laughing until it gets dark.

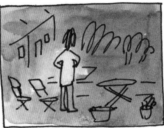

They go and do the washing-up.
I look at the night and wonder if I'll ever be able to relax properly again.

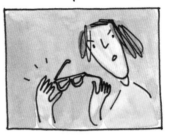

Later, I squash my glasses under the sofa by mistake.
'Damn!'

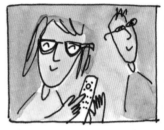

Bend them back into shape and they seem to fit better than they did before.
'I am winning at life again! Let's watch TV!'

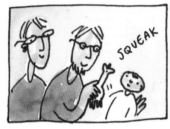

Tom's parents come down and look after James for the day.
'It's a giraffe, hello!'

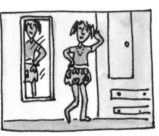

I dress up in a nice outfit to do errands.
'Me time!'

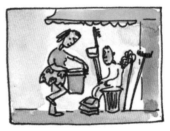

Go and buy a new bin.
'They're a bit stuck.'
'How about one of these? Save you bending over.'
'No thanks, I prefer normal dustpan and brushes.'
'Like getting down on the floor, eh? Heh heh.'
'Yep.'

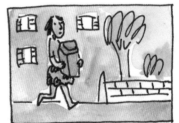

Carry the new bin home and think about how now I've got to throw the old bin in the bin. Infinity. Bin-finity?

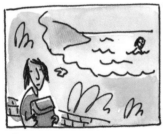

Then think about things I'm looking forward to doing when I've had the operation reversed:
Going swimming.

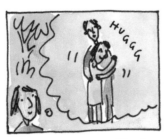

Hugging people without there being a bag of shit between me and them.

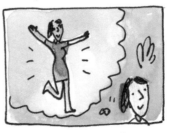

Wearing tight clothes.

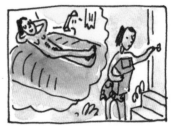

Being naked.
I <u>hate</u> being naked at the moment.

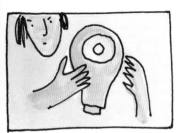

Some people have suggested giving the colostomy bag a name. FUCK THAT!

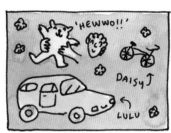

Same sort of people who give names to their cars and bikes and talk to cuddly toys.

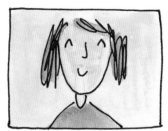

I prefer to call it: 'A FUCKING BAG OF SHIT.'

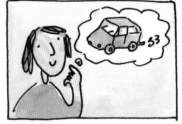

Actually, that's not far off what I used to call my old car. I miss it! Satsuma peel, receipts and shoes all over the floor, road trips to Yorkshire...

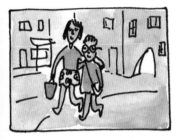

Before next chemo dose, blood-test machine is broken and there's a long wait to hear if I can have it or not. Me and Mum go to look for a garden to sit in.

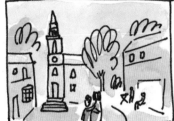

We wander about St James' churchyard in Clerkenwell. 'Lovely!'

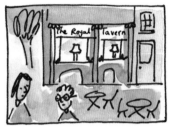

Then look for somewhere to have lunch. 'They're not open yet. Told me to "please leave the premises".' 'What? Poncy old gastropub. Didn't want to go there anyway.'

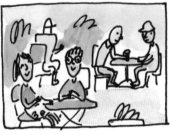

We find somewhere else. 'Always know a cafe is good if it's full of workmen.' 'Whatcha going to have?' 'Pulled pork bap.' 'Hehe.'

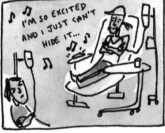

Blood is OK so have the next dose as planned. Surly bloke with lots of tattoos listens to Magic FM on his phone the whole time. So annoying! I'm too scared to ask him to turn it off.

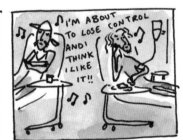

Another stringy old man next to him looks annoyed too. He's got some rice cakes in clingfilm and is eating them, crossly.

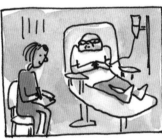

A nutritionist talks to a different man about diet. 'You need to be aiming for at least 5 fruits or veg a day.' 'Does jam count? I have jam every breakfast. What about Vimto? It's blackcurrant, isn't it?'

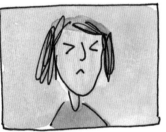

Can't believe I've got the same cancer as these ill old dudes.

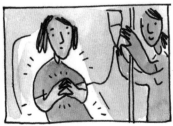

Nurses connect the second drug that I usually have. I start to feel really itchy.

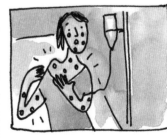

Suddenly get a weird rash. 'Mum! I'm covered in spots! Can you get a nurse?'

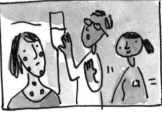

Lots of rushing about. 'Can you breathe OK?' 'Yep...' 'Blood pressure's normal.'

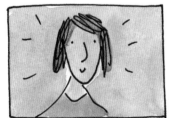

Given some more steroids and antihistamines and the rash goes as quickly as it appeared. 'Phew!'

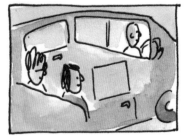

Tired out, we get a taxi home. The driver asks if we've had a nice day. 'Not really. Been in hospital having chemotherapy all afternoon.'

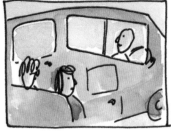

'Oh yeh? Wotcha got then, cancer?' ''Fraid so.' 'Ah dear. All my family's had it, they're all OK... Are you a believer?' ''Fraid not.'

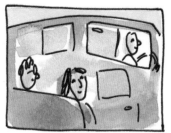

'Oh, you've gotta be a believer!' 'I like to keep an open mind.' Glad he doesn't ask me anything else about God. Enjoy telling him the whole story. 'My insides nearly burst!'

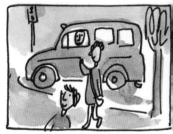

'Here you go then, ladies.' We give him a tip. 'Don't worry, you'll be alright, sweetheart.' 'Thanks, see ya!'

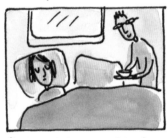

Really tired after this dose, with stomach cramps again. Tom brings me tomato soup.

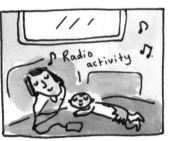

Codeine helps. Stay in bed all day listening to Kraftwerk.

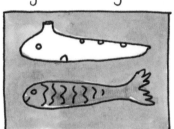

My dad comes to visit. He brings me an ocarina and a ceramic fish from Estonia.

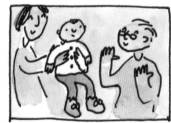

And some cute boots for James. 'So nice! What a trendy outfit!'

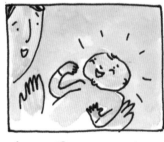

Later, James properly smiles at me for the first time. I think I feel happier than I've ever felt!

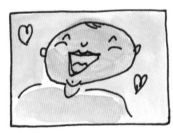

Then he smiles even more and half his mouth goes down on one side. So gorgeous!

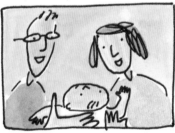

Tom and me try to make him smile again. 'Wa wa wa wooooo!' 'Come on, laddie, give us another.'

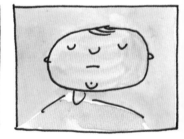

He doesn't like to waste them.

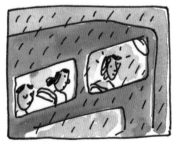

Go for a work meeting later in the week. Attack of chemo diarrhoea. Immodium doesn't work on me any more.

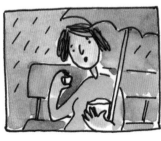

Eat a bag of marshmallows on a bench in Embankment Gardens so I don't explode in the meeting.

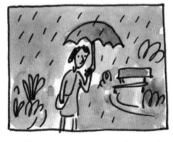

Then walk around the banana plants for a bit.

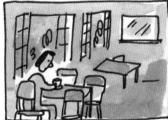

Wash the marshmallows down with a cup of tea at the garden cafe. Meditate for a bit until it's time to go.

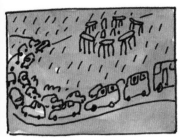

Drive to Taunton to Amy's wedding. Traffic slows down by Stonehenge so people can get a look at it.

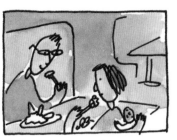

Pub at the B+B is just about to close when we arrive, they don't mind making us food.
I have cauliflower cheese and Tom has bangers+mash.
'Sausage weather again!'

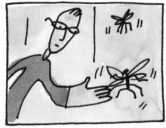

Our room is in a chalet round the back. There are a lot of daddy-long-legses about.
'Come on, dude, the door's over here.'

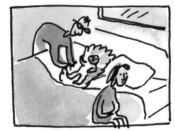

James has outgrown his travel-cot and we make a nest on a sheepskin between our pillows.
'Lovely and cosy.'
'I feel a bit sick.'

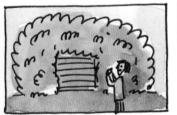

'Maybe it's just anxiety.'
'Mm, cheese and anxiety, not a good combo.'

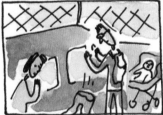

'And my chest hurts. I feel so paranoid, I'm convinced it's going to kill me. Everything else is so good it would balance things out if I died.'

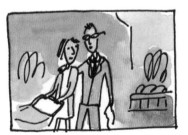

'Well I'm convinced it's not going to kill you. And everything's been so shit it would balance things out if you don't die.'

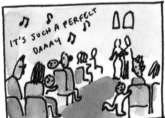

Fall asleep holding hands.
'I didn't just have a panic attack so as to avoid bringing things in from the car, you know.'
'Hehe, yeah right.'

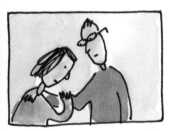

Before the wedding, see an interesting garage covered in a huge wig of ivy.
The only photo I manage to take before my phone battery runs out.

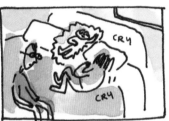

I forget to find out where the next B+B is before my phone dies, so Tom has to change into his suit on the way. Drops his trousers in a puddle.
'Shit!'

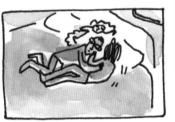

'Sorry I'm so disorganised.'
'S'alright.'
All ready to go.

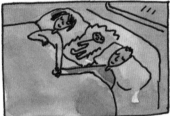

Excellent wedding. We sit at the back with the other people with children.
Good loud singing coming from Amy's actor friends.

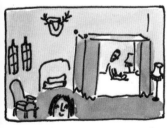

Next B+B is very grand. James looks tiny on the four-poster bed.
'I'm going to check out the bathroom.'

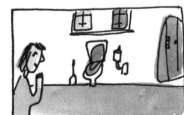

'It's practically bigger than our flat!'
Toilet in the middle of a big empty wall.

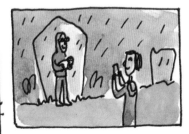

Stop at Avebury Stone Circle on the way home. Laugh about funny place names nearby.
'Say "Curry Wallop"!'

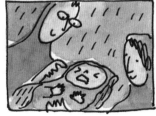

James hates the sudden cold, rainy weather.
'Sorry, lad, this lovely summer has led you to believe Britain is something that it isn't. 9 months of this now.'

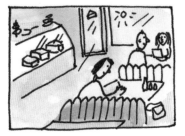
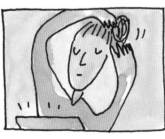
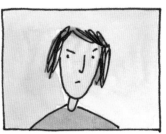
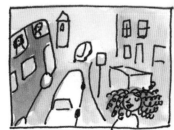

After a bloodtest, there's time before a doctor's appointment to sit in my new favourite cafe near the hospital and do some drawing. Stacks of ciabatta, sunlight streaming in.

Girl at the next table enjoys twisting her hair up into a knot.

I think: 'Alright, you've got an excellent big bun, no need to rub it in.'

On the way home, a girl waiting to cross the road tosses her curly hair about as she looks left, right, left again and right again. It goes everywhere and she loves it!

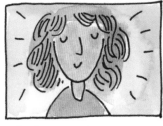
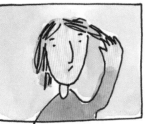
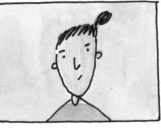
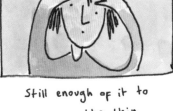

All being well, next year will be the year I have good hair. I'll be going for the Savoy Cabbage.

Rather than the Wilted Spinach.

I can just about put what's left of it into a very tiny aspirational ponytail. It looks a bit silly.

Still enough of it to cover up the thin patches.

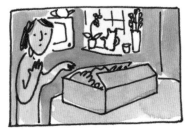
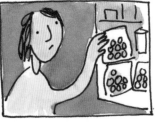
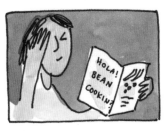
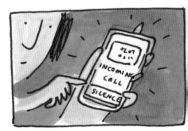

Speaking of vegetables, I decide it's time to cancel the veg box we get delivered. It always feels like a burden when it arrives- so big!

We never eat the potatoes fast enough and end up with hundreds.

Their leaflets are full of irritating over-friendly vegetable jokes.

They keep phoning to ask why I've left. It's like dumping a needy boyfriend. I never answer.

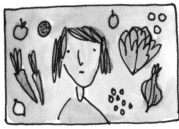
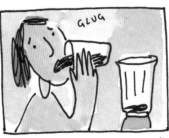
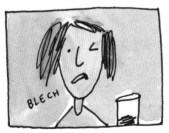
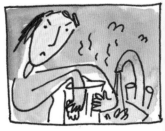

My oncologist told me I should try to eat 10 portions of fruit and veg a day. 10?!

Worried I'll have to spend the rest of my life anxiously necking horrible kale smoothies.
Do that a lot at the moment.

I can't pretend they're nice.

Hate washing the blender almost as much as I hate collapsing boxes. It's too heavy. With too many bits!

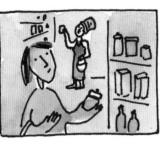

I try not to spend too much time in expensive health food shops.

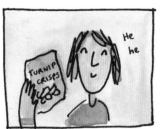

A while ago I wrote a poem about all the stuff you can buy in them. It went...

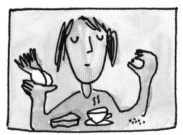

Pak choi, puy, chai, Yerba maté, quorn pie.

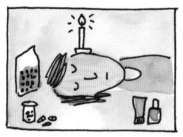

Goji, acai, Ayurveda, Hopi ear candle, Weleda.

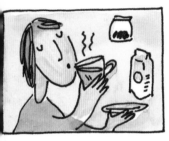

Blue-green algae, Birt and Tang, Oolong, Oatly, ylang ylang.

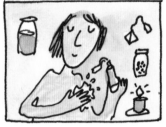

Agar agar, citronella, Tea Pig, arnica, chlorella.

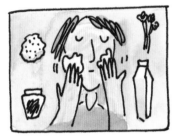

Dr Hauschka, spirulina, Rice cake, Provamel, verbena.

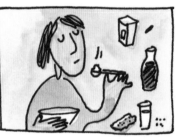

Flapjack, porridge, Pomegreat, Raisins, water, rooibos, date.

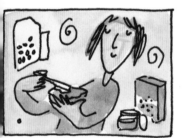

Cashew butter, fru-grain, Qi, Buckwheat, barley, pinto, pea.

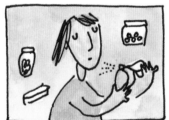

Mahi mahi, psyllium husk, Umeboshi plum, white musk.

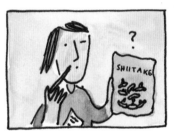

I couldn't think of an ending.

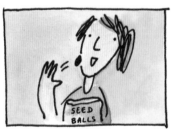

And still bought quite a lot of it.

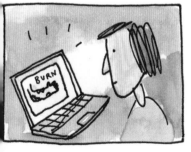

Have been researching the chemo drugs I'm on. Some derive from mustard gas. It was discovered to have cancer-suppressing properties during WW2.

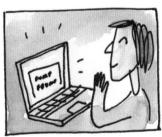

Some use acronyms FUMP and DUMP.

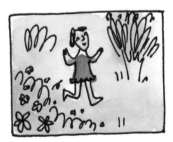

Lots come from plants, the periwinkle and the yew tree, for example.

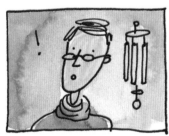

So stick that in your FUMP and smoke it, hippies!

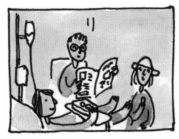

Penultimate chemo dose goes without a hitch. Leigh comes, we have popcorn and sushi again.

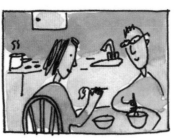

At home, me and Tom have been getting into Vietnamese cooking. 'About 4 of my 10 a day in this. And 7 garlic cloves.' 'Mm, delicious!'

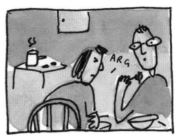

I get the usual symptoms, stomach cramps, diarrhoea etc.

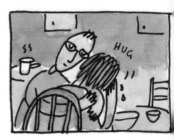

Weep into my noodle broth. 'It feels like it's never going to end.' 'Nearly there now, just gotta get through this last bit.'

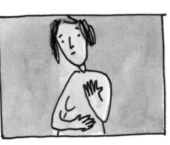

Spend a few days feeling depressed and lying in bed.

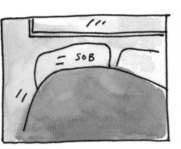

Completely under the covers. The best place to be.

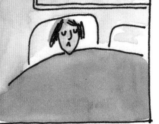

Can't be bothered to do anything.

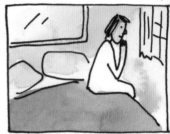

Even though it will be great not to have to go to hospital any more, I'm worried about not being closely monitored.

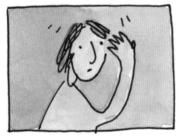

Anxious about every ache and pain. Headache : BRAIN METS*? *Mets = Metastasis= cancer spreading

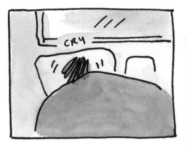

Stomach twinge: LIVER METS??

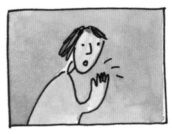

Slight cough: LUNG METS???

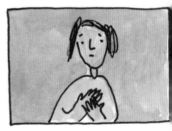

Palpitations: Permanent damage to my heart from the chemo????

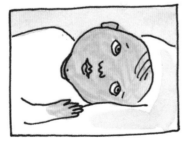

Am cheered up one morning by waking up to see James staring at my face instead of crying for food like he usually does.

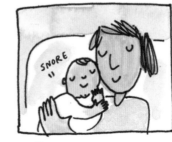

Most nights he wakes up at 3 or 4 and I take him out of his cot and put him next to me in bed.

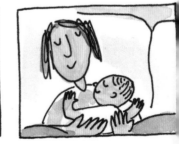

Those early mornings are the best!

He's almost too heavy now for me to sleep with him on my chest. Doze for a bit until it gets uncomfy

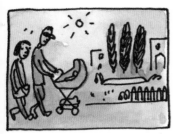

Beautiful early-autumn morning, powdery sunlight and haze. We take James for a walk around Bethnal Green.
'Ooh, look at those poplar trees.'

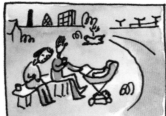

Coffees in Allen Gardens. More stomach cramps.
'I never liked that new office block, it ruined my view of the Gherkin when I lived in Stoke Newington.'
'Looks like a Pop-Tart.'

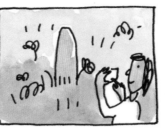

Take a photo of a bollard on its own in a load of grass.
'Heh, useless bollard!'

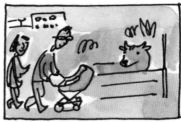

Stop at the city farm.
'Funny, isn't it, suddenly we keep going to places like the city farm, but James hasn't got a clue where he is!'
'What a calm cow.'

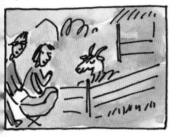

'That goat's got the same hair as your dad! Imagine it with a pint and a Kindle, so happy!'

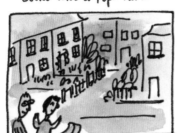

Carry on walking through Whitechapel.
'Victoria Cottages, cute! I guess it must all have been like this round here before the war.'
'Let's go down that alley.'

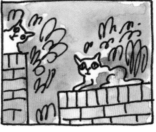

Some cats stare at us.

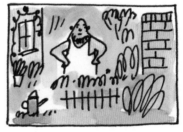

So does an old man.

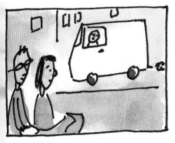

Bloke in a van stops to ask directions.
'You from round 'ere?'
'Um, no, sorry.'
Wish we were and could give directions.

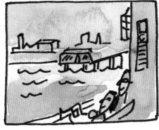

Walk all the way to Wapping and sit outside a pub by the river.
'Cor, look at everything, I love being alive!'

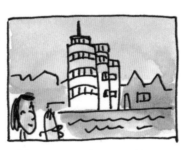

'I want to live in that art deco tower.
'We should walk there next time!'

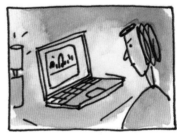

Later, I put the photo of the bollard I liked on the internet. People imply that it looks like a penis.
'It's not a penis! It's just a nice bollard.
Oh for fuck's sake.'

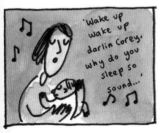

'Wake up wake up darlin Corey, why do you sleep so sound...'

Sing James all the folk songs I know.

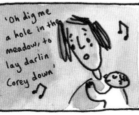

'Oh dig me a hole in the meadow, to lay darlin Corey down'

I need to learn some new ones, not about people dying, that don't make me cry!

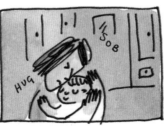

But the sad ones are my favourite.

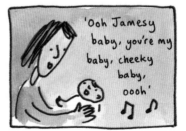

'Ooh Jamesy baby, you're my baby, cheeky baby, oooh'

Silly made-up songs are good.

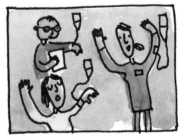

My dreams are still weird:
All the doctors have cancer
too and there's no hope
for any of us...

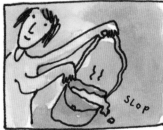

...shit porridge into
my handbag and am
happy about it...

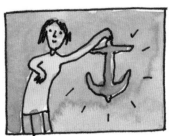

... then crap out a
massive rusty anchor.
Such symbolism!

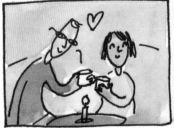

Also a nice normal one
about me and Tom
drinking whiskey sours
and being romantic.

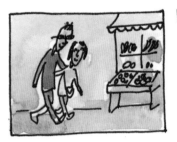

One morning, Tom's mum
looks after James and we
go to the veg shop. Feels like
we're on a date!

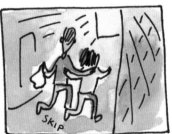

It's a treat to be out
together, just the
two of us.

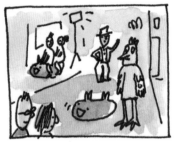

Some kind of music video
is being filmed in the street.
2-person space hoppers
and men waiting around
in droopy chicken suits.
'Eek, embarrassing.'

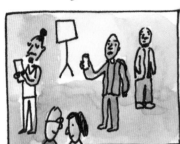

Tramps look unimpressed.
'Arg, I hate myself, I want
to tell the tramps I'm not
like these people.'
'Hehe, but you are just
like these people.'

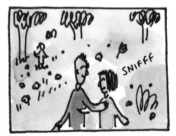

A new wild-flower
meadow's been planted
in the park.
'Mmm, smells like
the countryside.'

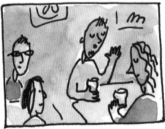

We go to a pub nearby.
Enjoy eavesdropping on
the couple next to us.
'Thing is, I always
get my way.
No compromise.'

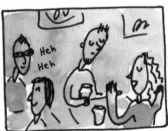

They're not really
listening to each other.
'Yah, I mean, I've always
been OBSESSED
with Epstein.'

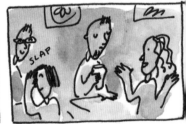

'There's literally, like, a
meadow? With all these
flowers in it? And there
were 2 prams?
And, like, a man?
Totally "WOW".'

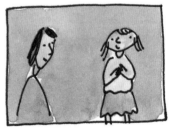

I've been finding that
when people say nice
things to me...
'I think you're a hero!'

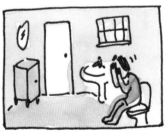

...it makes me cry.

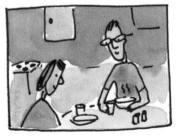

Especially when it's
Tom who says them.
'I'm so proud of you.'

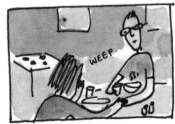

Still want people
to say nice things
all the same.

OCTOBER

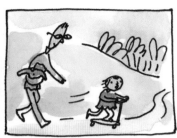

The little girl Tom looks after is about to start school.
'You can be Arabella and I'll be Lucinda.'
'Righto.'

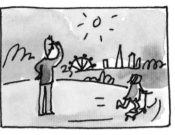

'Wow, Lucinda, look at the amazing view!'
'Yes, yes, I know. Come on, let's find the dinosaurs.'

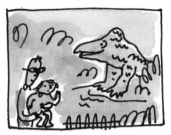

'Shh, Arabella, he might hear us.'
(Concrete dinosaurs in Crystal Palace Park.)

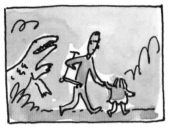

'Will I see you next week?'
'Not next week, you'll be at school, remember?'
'Oh yeah. I'll see you another time, then.'
'Yeh.'

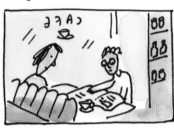

Me and Mum arrive early for my final dose of chemo. Sit in fave cafe and look at article about Japanese erotic art exhibition.

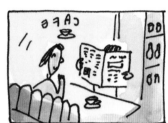

'You know, I don't think there are enough tentacles on that giant squid.'
'He he.'

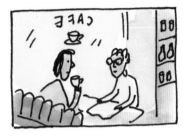

Talk about whether I should have my large intestine removed to lower the risk of cancer coming back.
'Well, I think about you every time I have a good shit.'

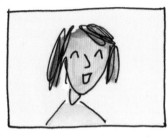

'Ha! Thanks, Mum.'

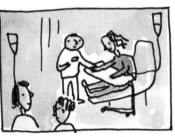

Dose is quick and easy. There's a woman with a shaky voice who keeps saying 'brilliant' and 'wonderful'.
'You'll be connected for 4 hours, my love.'

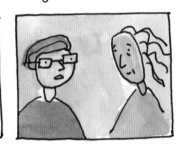

'Brilliant. thank you!'

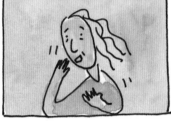

Her friend comes.
'You've got a bit of croissant on your cheek.'

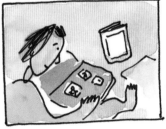

'Oh do I? Wonderful.'

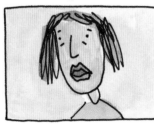

My lips are extra swollen afterwards.

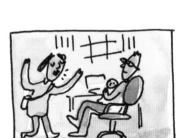

'Give us a kiss, boys!!'

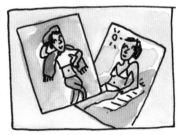

Look in photo albums for pictures of my old belly button.

Find a couple of nice ones from various holidays.

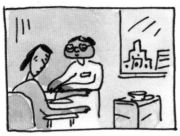

Go to get disconnected from the chemo pump and have my PICC line taken out. (AT LAST!) I'm nervous it'll hurt, and look out of the window.

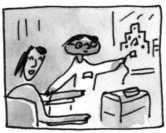

The nurse can tell and asks me about James. 'And how is baby?' 'oh he's fine, he's excellent!' (He takes it out and I don't even realise!)

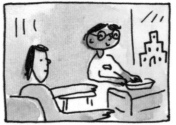

'Oh you've done it! That was easy!' He tells me that men cry more often than women at the end of their treatment. 'Because it's all over, you know?'

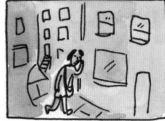

It doesn't feel like it's all over and I don't cry until I'm on my way home, on Bartholomew's close. Just a bit.

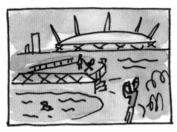

That afternoon, me, Tom and James go for a walk near East India Dock. Great view of the Millennium Dome. 'Like a giant beetle.'

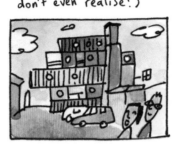

We check out some flats made out of shipping containers. 'Soooooo coooool.'

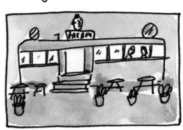

There's an authentic 40s diner shipped in from somewhere or other. 'Poor Fatboy would be turning in his grave at the size of this pastrami on rye!'

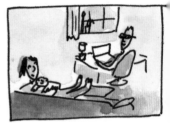

Don't do anything much celebratory in the evening. It's just nice being at home all together.

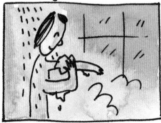

PICC line hole heals quickly. Feels great to give my left arm a good scrub.

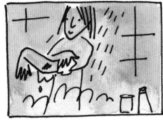

My left elbow has gone completely grey from not having been washed under the clingfilm. Whoops!

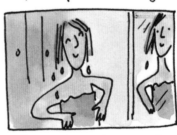

Almost back to normal.

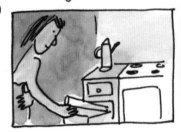

Put the clingfilm back in the kitchen drawer where it belongs!

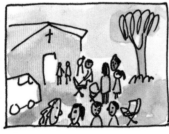

Go to a baby stuff jumble sale with Claire in Stoke Newington. 'Look at all these Stokey types.' 'Buggy overload.'

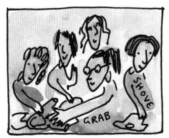

Everyone barges past each other, politely. 'Ooh, there's the Gap stuff.' 'Sorry, do you mind if I just...'

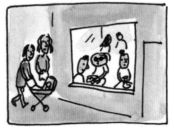

Lots of fashionable new cafes have opened since we lived here. All painted grey, without signs, full of hungover people eating eggs.

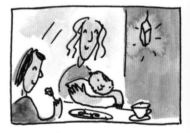

We find an emptyish not very trendy one. James stares at Claire's coffee cup for ages and smiles. 'Hehe, what's he looking at? Funny boy.'

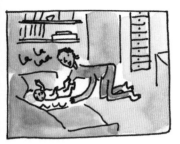

Hannah comes and has a good time singing with James.

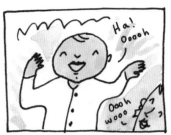

He's getting more smiley and responds to noises we make.

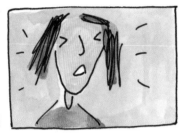

Mum calls him 'King of smiles'. 'You have to wait to be granted one.'

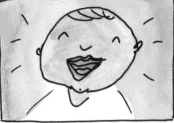

Just like the rising sun.

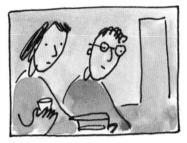

Go with Mum for another CT scan to check treatment has gone OK.

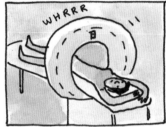

So nervous about the results that my bones hurt.

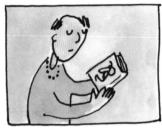

Some people suggest I got cancer because I'm 'holding on to pain.' 'Please, have this book, it will change your life!'

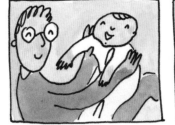

Would it help release some of my pain if I told you to 'FUCCKKK OFFFFF'??

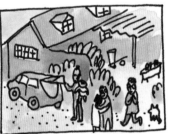

We go to my parents' for a week to recover from the treatment. 'My darlings!'

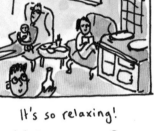

It's so relaxing! 'Pink wine, Tom? 'Ooh, yes please.'

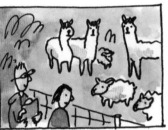

Take James to see the alpacas down the lane. 'Seems like the sheep are in charge.'

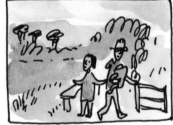

Tell him about all the other places. 'And this is where Granny fell in a ditch once...'

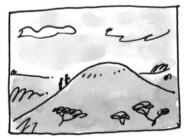

Go up the Trundle (an ancient hilltop fort). 'I love it up here so much. Me and Amy used to eat mini croissants, smoke fags and pretend to do the Riverdance at the top when we were teenagers.'

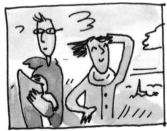

You can see all the way from Portsmouth to Brighton. 'If I die, scatter my ashes up here. And some by the sea. 'Okay.'

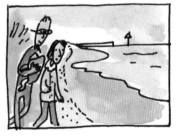
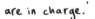

Walk all the way along Littlehampton West beach. 'What is it with those sandworms, what do they DO?'

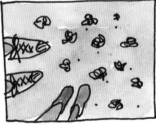

'Just dig holes and make wiggly piles of sand, I guess...' 'Shall we go back the way we came?' 'Yeh.'

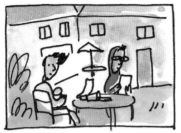

Have a windy lunch at the pub down the road from my parents'. 'This used to be a Cheddar-ploughman's-type pub...'

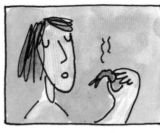

'But now you have to have stuff like prawn tempura.'

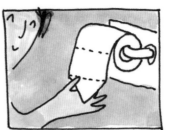

End of the loo roll folded into a point.

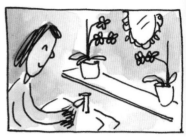

Orchids in the toilet.

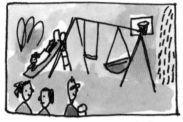

Go to see our friends in their new house near Brighton. 'Lovely willow tree!' 'I'm sliding down on my front!'

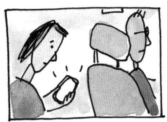

On the way home I get an email from my surgeon saying that I need another scan. 'Apparently my liver's changed colour. It might be nothing but they want to check.'

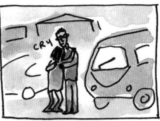

Stop in a supermarket car park. 'I don't think I can carry on being brave. I'm not strong enough for all this...' 'You are strong.'

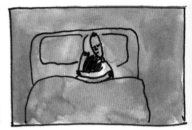

Scared.

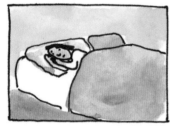

It's exhausting being anxious the whole time. Just want to lie in bed until I know what's going on.

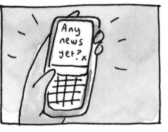

I lie to people about the results.

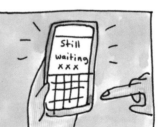

Because I can't face explaining it all again and again.

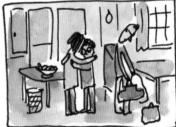

At the end of the week. 'Don't want you to go.' 'Don't want to go.'

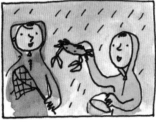

The following week we go to Southwold with Tom's family. Twins crabbing. 'It nearly pinched my finger!'

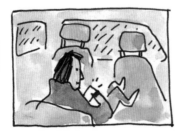

Me sheltering in the car.

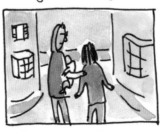

Tom points out places from his childhood. 'That's where I lay on the ground screaming after eating 20 Wham bars when I was about 8.'

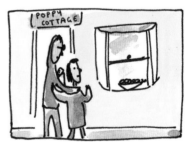

Practically every house seems to be for holiday lets. We play 'guess if it's a normal house or not.' 'Gotta be a holiday home, look at that bowl of stones.'

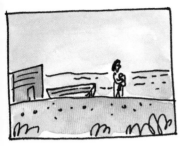

Day trip to Dunwich beach. I drive there with James and arrive before the walking party. Walk about feeling motherly.

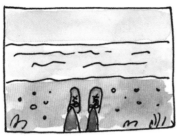

Look out to sea at where the sunken town ought to be. (Dunwich was a large Anglo-Saxon port that got washed away.)

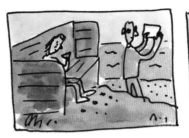

Old people eating sandwiches and taking photos on their iPads.

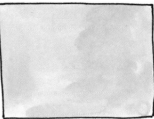

No clouds at all.

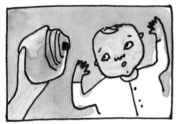

After fish + chip lunch, looking at pebbles with the twins.
'Look, this one's definitely interesting, stripey.'
'Ooh yes, that's a good one!'

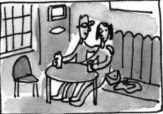

Later, kite flying.
'Watch out for the trees!'
'I want a go!! Waaa!.'
'Wow, so high!'

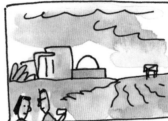

Me and Tom go to check out Sizewell B Nuclear Power Station.
'Did you get a good photo?'
'Yeh.'

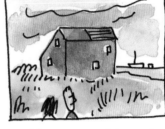

Admiring picturesque boat sheds at Walberswick.

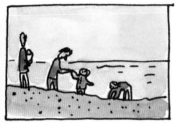

There's a bakery in Southwold where Tom gets me a pain au chocolat as big as James's head!

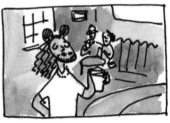

Walk along the promenade. A man who's just been kite-surfing does a handstand.

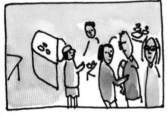

Go to a warm pub and talk about films we need to watch.
'Who's that guy, Warm Windows?'
'Wim Wenders?'
'Yeh, that's him.'

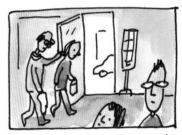

Kite-surfing guy arrives. He's wearing Mickey Mouse ears.
'I want to go to his parties.'
'Ha!'

On our last morning we go to the bakery cafe.
'That woman'd better not buy the last pain au chocolat!'

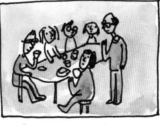

Everyone is very English about the communal table.
'Um, do you mind if we...'
'It's just I'm not sure I can move...'
'Ah, what about if we squeeze on the end?'
'Mm, don't know if...'

A man comes back who was sitting where we're sitting.
'Oh. They've cleared up my granola.'

'I was still eating that.'
'Oops.'

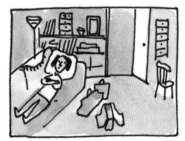

Arrive home. Feel depressed to be back in London, still without a scan result.

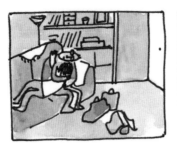

Long hug. My head feels like a pearl clamped safely in an oystershell.

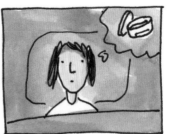

That night, I think about things that remind me of bad times. The smell of the geranium hand cream I had in hospital. (I used to love geranium body stuff.)

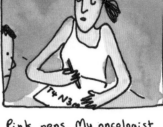

Pink pens. My oncologist used one to explain my diagnosis in Feb. She wrote upside down.

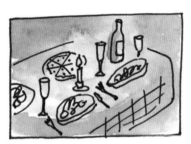

Trips to the Italian. It was always the closest place.

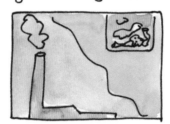

Think about my tumour, stored in a jar in a fridge somewhere.

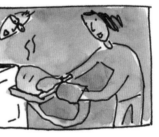

Or maybe it got burnt or lobbed in a bin.

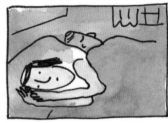

I sent some of my blood to researchers in Oxford. It's strange to think of pieces of my body hanging around elsewhere in the world.

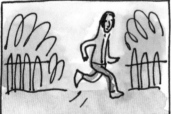

Next day, I go for a gentle jog. Got to start exercising every day (oncologist said). So unfit after months of inactivity!

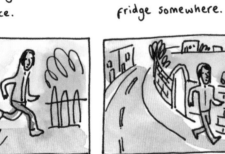

Go down empty streets, hoping no one will see me.

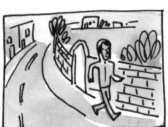

Later, I cook my first ever *ROAST*. 'Phoar, look at it! I've become a run and a roast on a Sunday bore!'

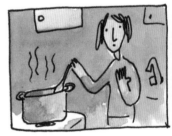

Make a huge pot of stock from the bones and forget I've got nothing to put it in.

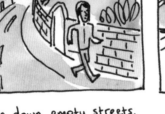

Hurricane St Jude rattles by outside. Can hear a bin flapping about.

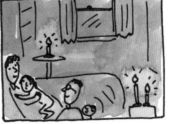

Still going at 6 in the morning. Our old-fashioned sash windows shake, evocatively.

Remember The Great Storm of 1987. Enjoyed the wuthering and candles in my parents' purple bedroom, aged 5.

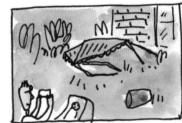

Tom takes James out and sends me pictures of the devastation. 'Gazebo hell!'

NOVEMBER

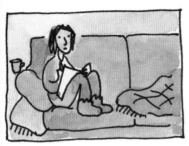

I've been finding that even though I write about things very openly in this comic...

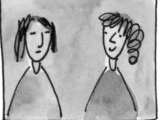

... and readily post personal stuff on the internet...

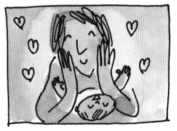

I don't actually want to talk about it all with very many people.
'Got any more hospital visits coming up?'
'Hope not.'

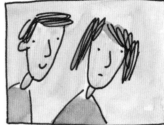

'So, how are you feeling now that treatment is over?'
'Oh, you know, anxious. I just want to forget about it altogether!'

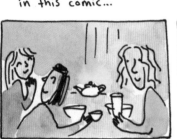

Have a nice evening out with Claire and our friend Hennie.
She's pregnant again.
'I knew it!'
'Ha ha, excellent!'

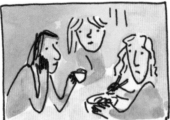

Having said I don't like talking about things, it's good to talk about things with them.
'Absolutely shitting it about the scan.'

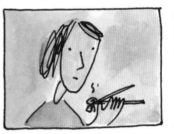

Sort of enjoy flippantly mentioning 'death'.
'If it's a bad result it'll mean more chemo, operations, might die etc.'

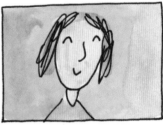

I think the trick is not to mention any of it to me unless I mention it first.

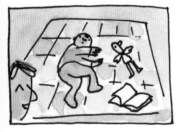

Stop myself panicking by madly tidying the flat...
'Gotta stop this nappies on the window sill situation!'

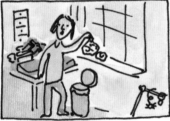

... by darning more jumpers...

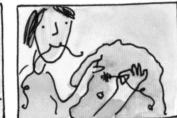

... and by reading articles.
'Urgh, when jellyfish die, their cells just blob together to make new jellyfish.'

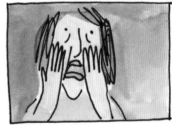

'Thousands of jellyfish can merge to make one giant jellyfish hundreds of feet across, some are the arse, some the skin, soooo grosss!!'

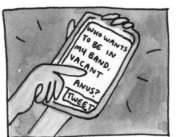

James is a good distraction too, of course. He can almost roll over now.
'Clever boy!'

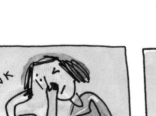

And can grab things purposefully.
'Ow!'

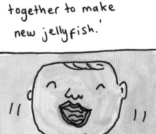

Very occasionally he laughs!

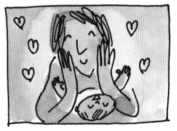

The best noise!

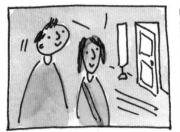

Meet Edwin and go to a comics fair.
'I read this comic about colonic irrigation the other day, it reminded me of you!'

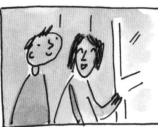

'What?! I thought I had the monopoly on colons!'

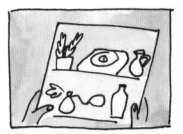

Buy a nice print (no name on it!).

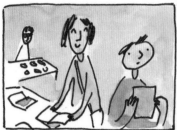

There's some cool stuff.
'A bum with eyes. Hmmm.'

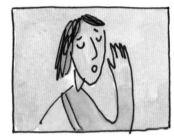

'So many comics start with things like, "Sometimes I feel like I don't exist..."'

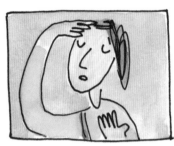

'Or, "Three cups of tea and I'm still sad".'

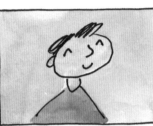

'We've all been there!'

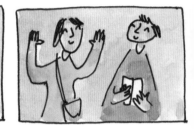

'Get some real problems for heaven's sake!'

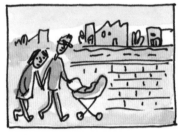

The next day, Tom, me and James go to find the art deco tower I saw across the river from Wapping.

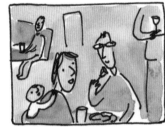

Roast dinner in a cosy pub, first.
"'Scuse me, you forgot my Yorkshire pudding.'
(Real problem.)

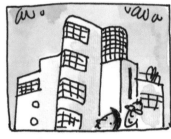

Tower is great in close-up, too.
'Phoar!'

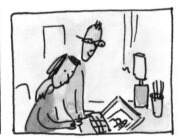

Look it up on the internet when we get home.
'Oh! Actually it was built in 1990 in the style of art deco. I still like it!'

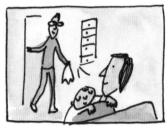

It's fireworks night.
'Just saw some when I went to the shop!'

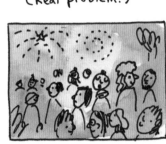

Last time I went to a firework display I got stuck in a crowd next to a man who kept saying 'disingenuous'.

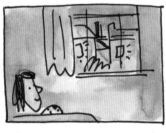

Can see more reflected in the windows of the derelict children's hospital down the street.

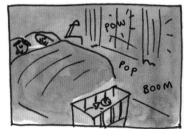

Maybe we'll go to some next year.

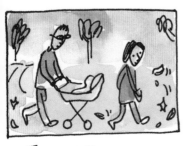

Tom and James come with me to the MRI scan.

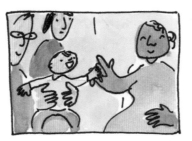

James makes friends with everyone in the waiting room.

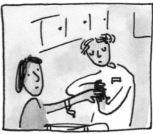

The nurse has trouble getting the cannula in my hand because my veins have been 'overused.'

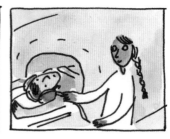

Ask for music this time.

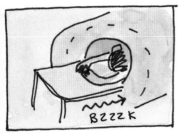

Forgot how claustrophobic it is.

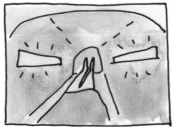

Try to keep my eyes closed.
If I do open them, down the tube looks like this.

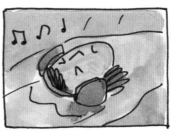

The MRI machine really needs a new chillout DJ. Awful 90s triphop with saxophones and scratching. Feel like I'm trapped in a coffin.

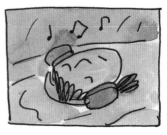

Whatever happened to whale song?? I guess then I'd feel like I'd been swallowed by a whale.

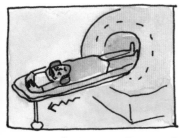

It played Samuel Barber's Adagio for Strings as I was slowly ejected. Seriously!

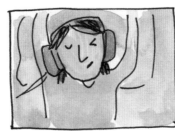

Imagine I'm the good guy that gets killed off in every crap short film ever made.

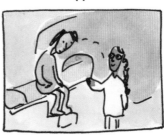

'Well done, dear— you lay so still we got some really clear pictures.'

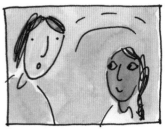

'Did you see anything? I know you're not meant to tell me.'
'We don't analyse the scans, I only know they got some good ones so the doctors can look.'

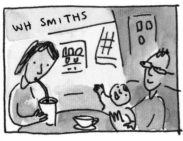

Have a choc-orange mochaccino with Tom and James in hospital Costa before we go.
'He really likes it in here, WH Smiths is so bright and colourful!'

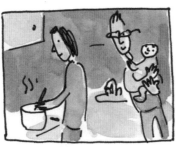

At home, make a banana curry for us. 'Mm, smells good!'

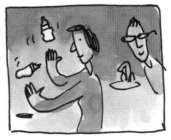

Later, sterilising bottles. 'I feel like Tom Cruise in that film where he makes cocktails.'
'You mean, Cocktail?'

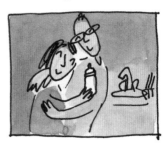

'Yes! Ha.'

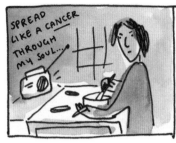

Another thing I've started to notice and dislike is when people use cancer as a metaphor for anything that spreads.

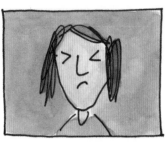

Like it's the worst thing in the world. As if I need reminding.

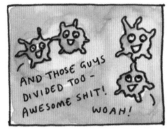

First of all, it's just lazy, easy, clichéd writing.

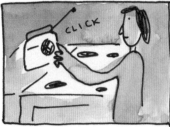

Second of all, it's inaccurate. Some cancers spread very slowly and can easily be contained.

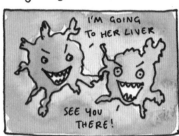

I also don't like the way cancer is described as 'evil' and 'malign', like the mutated cells have a villainous agenda.

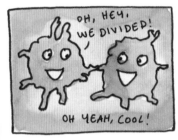

I find it easier to deal with if I just think of them as stupid, and doing what they're doing by accident.

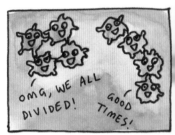

It seems more likely that my body can deal with them that way.

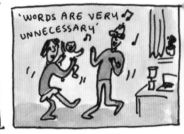

Hope I spoil their party.

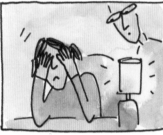

Hard not to worry about scan results the whole time. 'OH GODDD, I WANT IT TO BE CLEAR SO BADLY!'

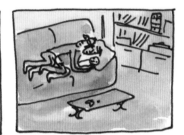

'What would you do without me?' 'Don't think about it.'

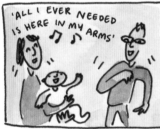

Cheer up and dance to Depeche Mode. 'He loves it!'

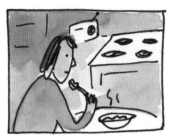

James laughs his head off at us. 'Let's try some Soft Cell on him tomorrow.'

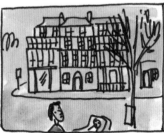

Next day, take James for a walk. We go past the derelict hospital. There's a plan to knock it down to make way for...

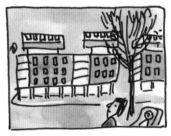

... Ugly, expensive, new builds. I wonder what would happen to the ghosts.

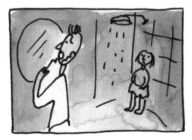

I hope they'd appear in the corners of brown-tiled wet rooms.

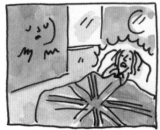

And press their faces through soft-touch purple walls. (That's what I'd do!)

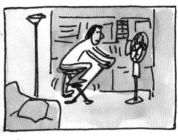

Hope the exercise bike will take my mind off things.

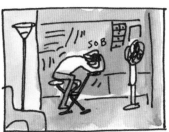

It doesn't work very well.

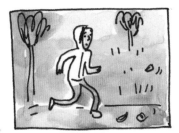

Try running about outside again.

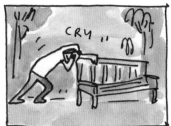

That doesn't work very well either. (Pretending to stretch.)

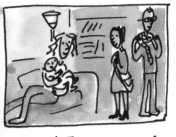

Me and Tom go for our first evening out together since James was born. Claire babysits.
'If he really won't sleep you have to rock him, "shush" him AND stroke his head.'

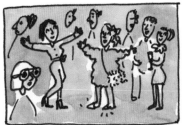

Meet Cesca, Adam and our friend Elinor at a club in Soho.
'Amazing onesie!'
'Wow, furry handbag!'
Friends distract away from anxiety much better than exercise.

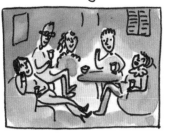

Laugh about things from the 90s.
'I was always a Lynx Aqua deodorant kinda guy.'
'I love the smell of that stuff! Mixed with Tipp-Ex and salt + vinegar crisps.'
'Mmm, such a turn-on.'

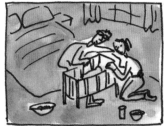

James went to sleep fine. We eat bowls of crisps, quietly.
'What a good boy.'

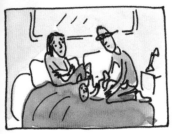

Next morning, expecting a call from the surgeon with the scan result.
'It must be bad news, he'd have phoned by now if it was all OK...'

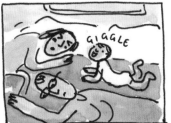

'They're probably just too busy to phone.'
James thinks my crying is really funny.

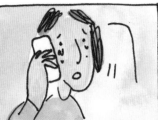

The surgeon phones.
'Hello? Yes, it's me...'

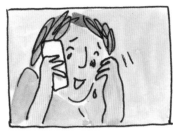

'It's clear?! Nothing at all? Oh! Thank you so much for phoning! Sorry to cry.'
(Floods of tears.)

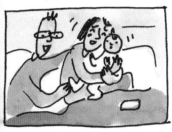

Sob and shake. James looks bewildered.
'I don't believe it!'
'Yesssss!'

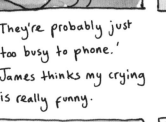
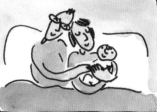
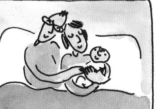

Calm down a bit.
'What shall we do to celebrate?'
'I dunno... go on the Greenwich cable cars?'
'Shall we have some tea first?'

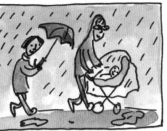

Change our minds about the cable cars and go out to get some noodles instead.

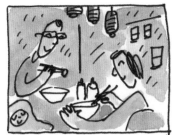

Talk about how we're both looking forward to normal times and eat summer rolls.
(Then have noodles.)

Thank you: All the doctors and nurses who kept me and James alive, and who continue to provide exceptional care. Tony Lacey at Penguin and my agent Elinor Cooper at Rochelle Stevens. Tweeps and kind people from the internet. My parents, Emma and Mike Tristram, and the rest of my tremendous family and friends. Most of all, Tom and James. As well as being quite unlucky I am very, very lucky.

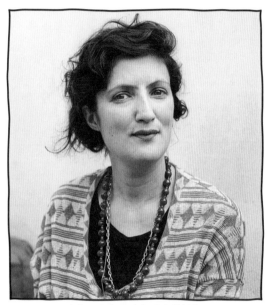

Author photograph by Jude Edginton

Matilda studied animation at the Royal College of Art and now lectures in drawing and moving image at Kingston University. She is a writer for children's TV (*The Adventures of Abney and Teal* and *Dipdap* for CBeebies) and her short films have screened at festivals internationally. Tom and Matilda's first picture book, *Santa's Beard*, is published by Walker Books. To see more of her work visit

www.mmaattiillddaa.com

VIKING

Published by the Penguin Group
Penguin Books Ltd, 80 Strand, London WC2R 0RL, England
Penguin Group (USA) Inc., 375 Hudson Street, New York, New York 10014, USA
Penguin Group (Canada), 90 Eglinton Avenue East, Suite 700, Toronto, Ontario, Canada M4P 2Y3
(a division of Pearson Penguin Canada Inc.)
Penguin Ireland, 25 St Stephen's Green, Dublin 2, Ireland (a division of Penguin Books Ltd)
Penguin Group (Australia), 707 Collins Street, Melbourne, Victoria 3008, Australia
(a division of Pearson Australia Group Pty Ltd)
Penguin Books India Pvt Ltd, 11 Community Centre,
Panchsheel Park, New Delhi – 110 017, India
Penguin Group (NZ), 67 Apollo Drive, Rosedale, Auckland 0632, New Zealand
(a division of Pearson New Zealand Ltd)
Penguin Books (South Africa) (Pty) Ltd, Block D, Rosebank Office Park,
181 Jan Smuts Avenue, Parktown North, Gauteng 2193, South Africa

Penguin Books Ltd, Registered Offices: 80 Strand, London WC2R 0RL, England

www.penguin.com

First published 2014
001

Copyright © Matilda Tristram, 2014

The moral right of the author has been asserted

Set in Kidprint
Designed by Alison O'Toole
Colour reproduction by Altaimage, London
Printed in China

A CIP catalogue record for this book is available from the British Library

ISBN: 978-0-241-00415-9

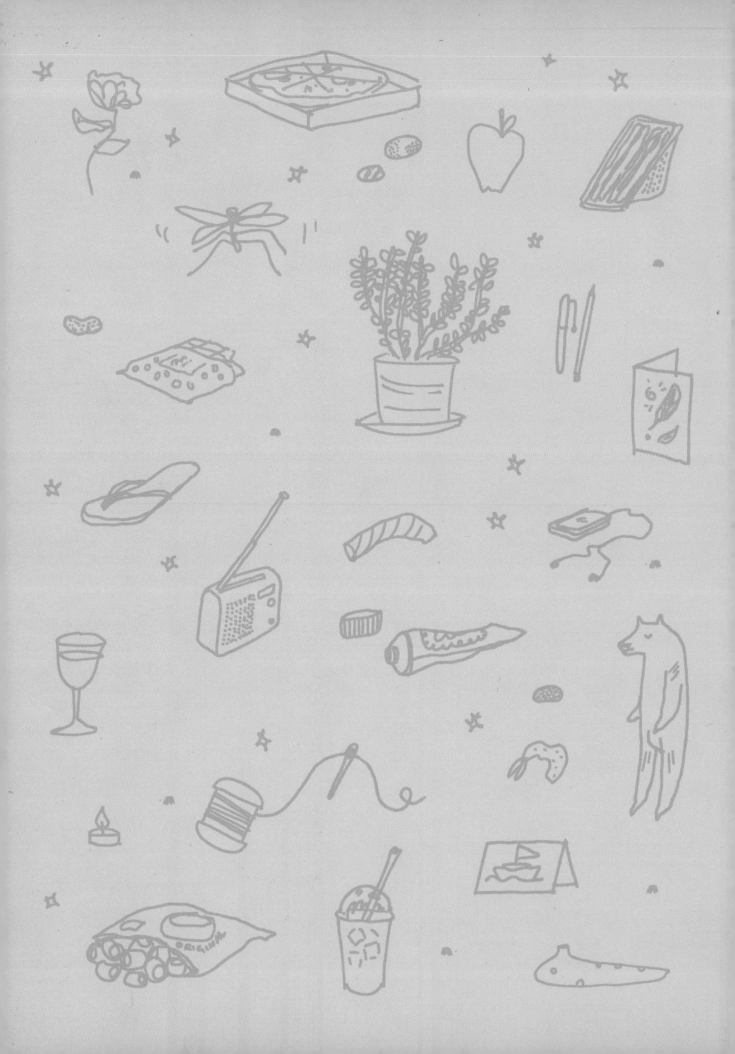